Neuroanatomy and Neurophysiology
A Review

NEUROANATOMY AND NEUROPHYSIOLOGY: A REVIEW

Jonathan Stuart Citow, M.D.
Clinical Assistant Professor
Department of Neurosurgery
University of Chicago Medical Center
Chicago, Illinois

Robert L. Macdonald, M.D., Ph.D.
Associate Professor
Department of Neurosurgery
University of Chicago Medical Center
Chicago, Illinois

Foreword by Bryce Weir, O.C., M.D.

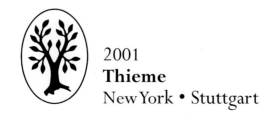

2001
Thieme
New York • Stuttgart

BS

The author and the publisher would like to thank the following companies for their financial support of this book:

Medtronic Sofamor Danek
Anspach Companies
DePuy AcroMed, Inc., a Johnson & Johnson company
Synapse Medical, LLC
Allegiance Healthcare Corporation
Bayer Corporation
BrainLAB USA

Thieme New York
333 Seventh Avenue
New York, NY 10001

Neuroanatomy and Neurophysiology: A review
Jonathan Stuart Citow
Robert L. Macdonald
Editorial Assistant: Diane Sardini
Director, Production and Manufacturing: Anne Vinnicombe
Production Editor: Becky Dille
Marketing Director: Phyllis Gold
Sales Manager: Ross Lumpkin
Chief Financial Officer: Peter van Woerden
President: Brian D. Scanlan
Cover Designer: Kevin Kall
Designer: Karin Badger
Compositor: Prepare, Inc.
Printer: G. Canale

5 4 3 2 1

TNY ISBN 1-58890-054-1
GTV ISBN 3-13-129221-0

Table of Contents

Foreword

The best books are those which take from the reader the least amount of time and money in return for the most information. Dr. Citow and colleagues have done yeoman work in distilling the vast corpus of clinical neuroscience into this concise, yet readable book. The illustrations portray essential information. Young neurosurgeons preparing for the hurdles for professional examinations will find this to be a most valuable aid. I suspect that those who use it and become familiar with its contents will continue to browse through it as the years go by to refresh their memories. All those involved in the care of patients with neurological diseases will read this work to their advantage. It is remarkable that Dr. Citow had the ability to write this book while still in his residency. Future residents will have reason to be grateful for his industry.

Bryce Weir, O.C., M.D.
Maurice Goldblatt Professor of Surgery and Neurosurgery
The University of Chicago
Chicago, Illinois

Preface

The neurosciences are an ever changing field, continuously evolving as information provided by more advanced research techniques is used to update and occasionally replace current concepts. Our knowledge of the innumerable connections and interactions in the nervous system is constantly growing, though the basic framework remains stable. This anatomy book draws its information from some of the classic texts as well as some more recent sources. Because most students of neuroanatomy do not have the well-needed time to delve deeply into the more intricate details of the nervous system, I have attempted to organize the more relevant points in a concise and easily referable manner. This book is certainly not intended to replace the more comprehensive texts that I have used as references, though it should provide its audience with a comfortable place to start.

Jonathan Stuart Citow, M.D.

References

Handbook of Neurosurgery, 3rd Edition. Greenberg MS. Lakeland, FL: Greenberg Graphics, Co., 1996.

Neurological Surgery, 4th Edition. Youmans JR (Ed.). Philadelphia, PA: W.B. Saunders, Inc., 1994.

Principles of Neurology, 5th Edition. Adams RD, Victor M. New York: McGraw Hill, 1993.

Diagnostic Neuroradiology. Osborne AG. St. Louis, MO: Mosby, 1994.

Neuroradiology, 3rd Edition. Ramsey RG. Philadelphia, PA: W.B. Saunders, Co., 1994.

Basic Neuroscience, 2nd Edition. Guyton AC. Philadelphia, PA: W.B. Saunders, Co., 1992.

Principles of Neural Science, 3rd Edition. Kandel ER, Schwartz JH, Jessel TM (Eds.). Norwalk, CT: Appleton & Lange, 1991.

Aids to the Examination of the Peripheral Nervous System. Tindall B. London: W.B. Saunders, Co., 1986.

Atlas of Human Anatomy, 7th Edition. Netter FH. Summit, NJ: CIBA-Geigy, 1994.

Clinically Oriented Anatomy, 3rd Edition. Moore KL. Baltimore, MD: Williams & Wilkins, 1992.

Core Text of Neuroanatomy, 4th Edition. Carpenter MB. Baltimore, MD: Williams & Wilkins, 1991.

Cranial Nerves: Anatomy and Clinical Comments. Wilson-Pauwels L. Hawthorne, Ontario: B.C. Decker, Inc., 1988.

Dedication

I wish to dedicate this book to my 15 month-old son Benjamin who everyday teaches me as much as I do him.

JSC

Acknowledgments

I wish to thank Loch Macdonald for his editing help and anatomy lectures. I wish to thank Lydia Johns for her wonderful artwork and killer sense of humor. I wish to thank my partners Sheldon Lazar and Jeffery Karasick for helping me to find time for this project. Most of all, I wish to thank my wife Karen for all of the behind the scenes laboring that enables endeavors like this to succeed.

Jonathan Stuart Citow, M.D.

ANATOMY

I. MENINGES

A. General—the brain and spinal cord are covered by three membranes collectively named the meninges. These layers from superficial to deep are the dura, arachnoid, and pia. The meninges help to protect the neural structures and also have circulatory functions (venous sinuses in the dura) (**Fig. A–1**).

B. Dura mater—literal translation is "hard mother". The intracranial dura has two layers: the periosteal layer and the meningeal layer. The periosteal layer does not extend caudal to the foramen magnum, thus the spinal dura has one layer. The spinal dura ends at S2, and the filum terminale continues as the **coccygeal ligament**. The spinal cord ends at L1/2 (in adults). Certain parts of the dura contain large low-pressure venous blood vessels between the dural layers **(dural sinuses)** that serve to conduct cerebral venous blood back toward the heart.

C. Arachnoid mater—thin avascular membrane adjoining but not tightly bound to the dura with filaments extending through the subarachnoid space and connecting to the pia. These gentle filaments cause the subarachnoid space to look similar to a spider web, thus the name *arachnoid* derived from the Greek word *arachne* meaning spider. The subarachnoid space contains the cerebral spinal fluid. Since the arachnoid is poorly adherent to the dura, blood may collect between these layers causing a **subdural hematoma**. Blood between the dura and the skull is an **epidural hematoma**.

D. Pia mater—contains an intimal layer (avascular, receives nutrients from the CSF and the neural tissue) and an epipial layer (continuous with the arachnoid trabeculae, absent over the convexities).

E. Falx cerebri—dural extension forming a divider between the two cerebral hemispheres.

F. Tentorium cerebelli—dural extension forming a boundary between the cerebellum and the cerebrum.

G. **Dentate ligaments**—connect the epipia to the dura and lie on the lateral surface of the spinal cord **between the ventral and dorsal roots**.

H. Filum terminale—an extension of epipia extending from the conus medullaris at the distal end of the spinal cord.

I. Virchow-Robin spaces—the spaces between the blood vessels and the surrounding sheath of arachnoid and pia where they enter the brain and spinal cord.

J. Blood supply—the **anterior meningeal artery** is from the ophthalmic artery. The **middle meningeal artery** is from the maxillary branch of the external carotid artery. The **posterior meningeal artery** is supplied by the occipital artery and the vertebral artery.

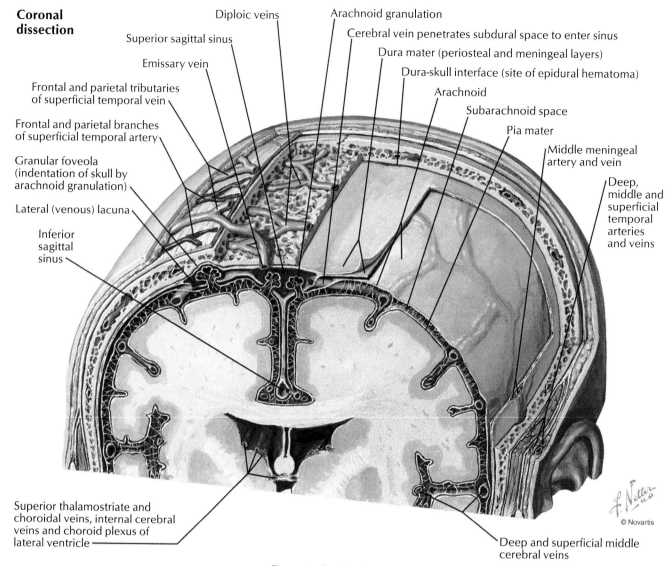

Coronal dissection

Diploic veins

Superior sagittal sinus

Emissary vein

Frontal and parietal tributaries of superficial temporal vein

Frontal and parietal branches of superficial temporal artery

Granular foveola (indentation of skull by arachnoid granulation)

Lateral (venous) lacuna

Inferior sagittal sinus

Arachnoid granulation

Cerebral vein penetrates subdural space to enter sinus

Dura mater (periosteal and meningeal layers)

Dura-skull interface (site of epidural hematoma)

Arachnoid

Subarachnoid space

Pia mater

Middle meningeal artery and vein

Deep, middle and superficial temporal arteries and veins

Superior thalamostriate and choroidal veins, internal cerebral veins and choroid plexus of lateral ventricle

Deep and superficial middle cerebral veins

© Novartis

Figure A–1   Meninges.

K. Innervation—the **supratentorial dura is innervated by the trigeminal nerve** (V1, anterior fossa; V2, middle fossa; and V3, mastoid air cells and posterior middle fossa). The **infratentorial dura (posterior fossa) is innervated by the upper cervical roots and the vagus nerve**.

L. Embryology—the pia, arachnoid, glia, ependyma, and neural parenchyma are formed from ectoderm. The **dura (posterior fossa) and blood vessels are formed from mesoderm**.

II. CEREBROSPINAL FLUID

A. Functions—the cerebrospinal fluid (CSF) removes waste, carries nutrition to the brain, is involved with regulation of various brain functions, neurotransmitters, paracrine and endocrine effects, and cushions the brain. Also, hypothalamic hormones are secreted in the CSF and transported by the ependymal cells into the hypophyseal portal system.

B. Contents—the CSF compared with plasma has similar osmolarity (295 mosm/L) and Na^+; **increased Cl^- and Mg^{++}; and decreased K^+, Ca^{++}, uric acid, and glucose.** Normal CSF glucose is 45 to 80 mg/dL ($\frac{2}{3}$ the serum value). Normal CSF protein is <45 mg/dL.

C. Volume—the total volume in the average 70-kg human is 150 mL, with 25 mL in the ventricles. 450 mL is produced each day.

D. Production—seventy percent of the CSF is secreted by the choroid plexus, 18% is capillary ultrafiltrate, and 12% is from metabolic water production. CSF production is an **active process** requiring the Na^+/K^+ ATP pump, with Na^+ being secreted into the subarachnoid space and water following it there from the blood vessels. CSF production is **decreased by carbonic anhydrase inhibitors (acetazolamide) and norepinephrine (NE)**. It is **increased by volatile anesthetics and CO_2**. It is also controlled by the raphe nuclei which send axons with serotonin to the periependymal vessels.

E. Arachnoid granulations—contain numerous arachnoid villi. They are most numerous around the superior sagittal sinus. They function as a **pressure-dependent one-way valve**, with collapsing tubules that transmit CSF when the intracranial pressure (ICP) is 3 to 6 cm H_2O greater than venous pressure. The arachnoid granulation cells transmit the CSF in giant cytoplasmic vacules by bulk flow into the venous sinuses.

F. Histology—the choroid plexus consists of a single layer of cuboidal epithelial cells surrounding blood vessels. The choroid is located in the caudal roof of the fourth ventricle (inferior medullary velum and lateral recess to the foramen of Luschka), the posterior roof of the third ventricle, and the floors of the bodies and the roofs of the temporal horns of the lateral ventricles.

G. Normal CSF cell count—less than 5 lymphocytes, and no PMNs or RBCs. The RBCs in a traumatic tap should be increased 700 RBC/1 WBC.

H. **Froin's syndrome**—due to loculation of the lumbar CSF. The CSF protein is increased (up to 1000mg/2L) and fibrinogen is present.

I. Intracranial pressure (measured in the lumbar cistern)—10 to 15 cm H_2O in adults (3 to 6 cm H_2O in children) when supine and 20 to 30 cm H_2O when sitting.

J. **Monro-Kellie doctrine**—the skull has a fixed volume that is filled up with brain tissue (1400 mL), blood in arteries and veins (150 mL), and CSF (150 mL). The added volume of a foreign body (tumor, hemorhage, etc.) forces removal of normal inhabitants of the skull. As the intracranial pressure increases, first the CSF leaves, than the venous blood, finally arterial blood and brain tissue (brain herniation).

K. Assessing CSF leakage—check for β-**transferrin**. It is only made in the CSF.

III. BRAIN BARRIERS

A. Blood brain barrier (BBB)—formed by the **capillary endothelial tight junctions** (mainly), pinocytic activity in the endothelial cells, and the astrocytic foot processes.

B. Molecular movement across the BBB—occurs by **diffusion** (H_2O), **carrier-mediated transport** (D-glucose, amino acids), and **active transport**. L-Glucose is not transported. Protein-bound molecules do not cross. These barriers are highly permeable to H_2O, CO_2, O_2, and lipid-soluble substances such as ETOH, barbiturates, heroin, and anesthetic agents. They are slightly permeable to ions such as Na^+, Cl^-, and K^+. They are impermeable to plasma proteins and large organic molecules.

C. **Circumventricular organs**—where the BBB is absent due to the presence of fenestrated capillaries.

   1. **Pineal gland**—produces melatonin and is involved with circadian rhythms.

   2. **Subforniceal organ**—lies between the interventricular foramen, connected to the choroid plexus, and may be involved with body fluid regulation.

3. **Subcommissural organ**—the only circumventricular organ with an intact BBB. Its function is unknown.

4. **Organum vasculosum of the lamina terminalis**—the outlet for hypothalamic peptides and may serve to detect peptides, amino acids, and proteins in the blood.

5. **Median eminence of the hypothalamus**—where the hypothalamic-releasing factors are released.

6. **Neurohypophysis**

7. **Area postrema**—the **only paired circumventricular organ.** It is located in the floor of the fourth ventricle and is a chemoreceptor that induces emesis when stimulated by digitalis or apomorphine.

D. Blood-CSF barrier—formed because the choroid cuboidal epithelium has tight junctions, although the blood vessels there have fenestrated capillaries.

IV. BLOOD SUPPLY TO THE BRAIN

A. General—the brain weighs 1500 g (2% of the body weight), but it receives **17% of the cardiac output (CO)** and uses **20% of the body's oxygen**.

B. Cerebral blood flow (CBF)—normally **50 mL/100 mg/min**.

C. **Ischemic penumbra**—area where there is decreased blood flow **8 to 23 mL/100 mg/min** that permits the neurons to survive but not function. At less than 8 mL/100 mg/min, the neurons die.

D. Vascular supply to the brain—variable and depends on several leptomeningeal anastomoses, many of which are from the external carotid circulation. The **anterior circulation** refers to blood flow reaching the brain via the internal carotid arteries, whereas the **posterior circulation** refers to blood flow from the vertebral and basilar arteries.

E. External carotid artery (ECA)—smaller than the internal carotid artery (ICA) and has eight major branches (SALFOPS Max) (**Fig. A–2**).

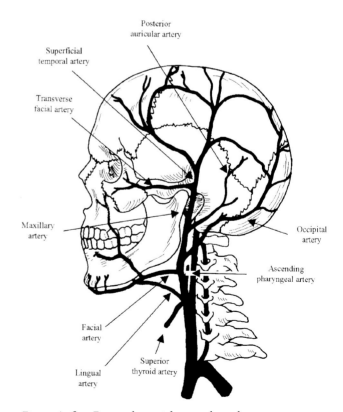

1. Superior thyroid artery—supplies the larynx and upper thyroid (the inferior thyroid and the isthmus are supplied by the thyrocervical trunk).

2. Ascending pharyngeal artery—supplies the nasopharynx, oropharynx, middle ear, CN IX, X, and XI, and the meninges. It anastomoses with vertebral artery branches.

3. Lingual artery—supplies the tongue and the floor of the mouth.

Figure A–2   External carotid artery branches.

4. Facial artery—supplies the face, palate, and lips. The angular branch anastomoses with the orbital branch of the ophthalmic artery.

5. Occipital artery—supplies the posterior scalp, upper cervical musculature, and posterior fossa meninges. It anastomoses with the vertebral artery.

6. Posterior auricular artery—supplies the pinna, external auditory canal, and scalp.

7. Superficial temporal artery—supplies the scalp and ear.

8. Internal maxillary artery—supplies the deep face and gives off the middle meningeal artery. It anastomoses with the inferior lateral cavernous sinus trunk and the ophthalmic artery through ethmoidal branches.

F. Internal carotid artery (ICA)

1. Cervical segment—no branches and lies posterolateral to the ECA in the neck.

2. Petrosal/intraosseus segment—travels through the carotid canal of the petrous temporal bone.

(a) Caroticotympanic branch—supplies the middle and inner ear (it may have an abberant course across the hypotympanium forming a pulsatile mass) and anastomoses with the anterior tympanic branch of the maxillary artery.

(b) Vidian artery (also called the artery of the pterygoid canal)—goes through the foramen lacerum and the vidian canal to anastomose with the ECA.

(c) A persistent stapedial artery from the ICA can form the middle meningeal artery if no foramen spinosum is present.

3. Intracavernous segment (**Fig. A–3**)

(a) **Meningohypophyseal trunk** (posterior trunk)

(i) **Tentorial artery (of Bernasconi and Casinari)**—supplies the mass of the tentorium.

(ii) **Inferior hypophyseal artery**—supplies the posterior pituitary capsule.

(iii) **Dorsal meningeal artery**—supplies CN VI and part of the clivus.

(b) Inferior cavernous sinus artery (lateral trunk)—supplies the inferolateral cavernous sinus wall and region of the foramen ovale and spinosum.

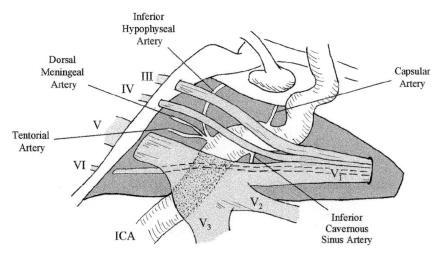

Figure A–3   Cavernous sinus ICA branches.

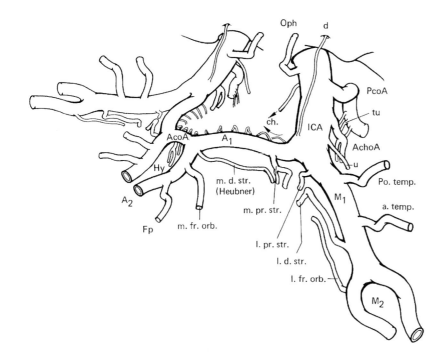

Figure A–4   An illustration of the classical anterior portion of the Circle of Willis and perforating arteries. The arteries are abbreviated as follows: ophthalmic (Oph), dural (d), chiasmatic (ch), posterior communicating (PcoA), tuberomammillary (tu), anterior choroidal (AchoA), uncal (u), middle cerebral artery (M_1 segment) superior, and inferior trunk (M_2), polar and anterior temporal (Po, a. temp.), lateral proximal and distal striate (l. pr. str., l. d. str.), A_1 segment (A_1), medial proximal striate (m. pr. str.), medial distal striate (m. d. str.), or Heubner's, anterior communicating (AcoA), hypothalamic (Hy), A_2 segment (A_2), medial fronto-orbital (m. fr. orb.), lateral fronto-orbital (l. fr. orb.), and fronto-polar (Fp) arteries.

    (c) McConnel's capsular artery (medial trunk)—present in 28% of the population and supplies the anterior and inferior pituitary capsule.

4.   Intradural segment/supraclinoid ICA (**Fig. A–4**)

    (a) Ophthalmic artery—rarely arises in the cavernous sinus. It usually lies inferior to the optic nerve. In the optic canal it is lateral and then crosses superomedially over the optic nerve in the orbit to supply the globe by way of the central retinal artery and the ciliary arteries. It supplies the orbit along with a minor contribution from the infraorbital branch of the maxillary artery that anastomoses with it. In 0.5% of cases, the ophthalmic artery arises from the middle meningeal artery and thus may result in blindness after embolization if not detected. Aneurysms arise from the superior wall of the ICA distal to the origin of the ophthalmic artery and point upward against the optic nerve.

    (b) Superior hypophyseal arteries—several small arteries arising from the inferomedial portion of the intradural ICA that course beneath the optic nerve to **supply the pituitary stalk, tuber cinereum, anterior lobe of the pituitary, and inferior surface of the chiasm**. These arteries anastomose with those from the contralateral side and the inferior hypophyseal arteries to form the **hypophyseal portal system**. Aneurysms arise from this area and point inferiorly and medially.

    (c) Posterior communicating artery (PCOM)—arises from the inferolateral wall of the ICA and courses posterolaterally above the oculomotor nerve to join the posterior cerebral artery (PCA). Fifty percent of PCOMs have variations such as absence, hypoplasia, duplication, and triplication.

        (i) **Fetal-type PCOM**—occurs when the diameter of the vessel is the same as the posterior cerebral artery (PCA). It occurs unilaterally in 20% and bilaterally in 8% of the population (**Fig. A–5**).

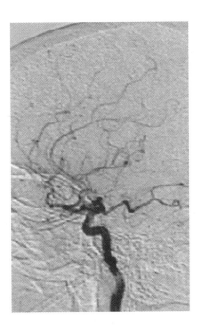 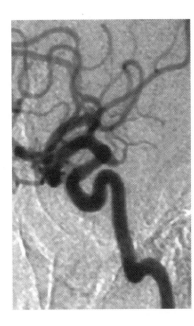

Figure A–5   Persistent fetal PCOM artery; angiogram demonstrates filling of the posterior circulation through the PCOM artery.

Figure A–6   PCOM artery infundibulum; angiogram demonstrates the vessel emerging from the tip of a pyramidal dilation.

(ii)   **Infundibulum**—a pyramidal base 3 to 4 mm in diameter at the ICA junction with the PCOM arising from the apex. It is detected in 10% of PCOMs (**Fig. A–6**).

(iii) Usually seven perforators are evenly distributed along the PCOM and course superomedially to **supply the posterior hypothalamus, anterior thalamus, posterior limb of the internal capsule (IC), and subthalamus**. The largest perforator terminates between the mamillary bodies and the optic tract and is called the **anterior thalamoperforating artery**.

(iv) Aneurysms—usually arise from the posterior wall of the carotid artery just distal to the take-off of the PCOM and point posteriorly toward the oculomotor nerve. The PCOM is found on the inferomedial side of the aneurysm, whereas the anterior choroidal artery is superior or superolateral to the aneurysm.

(d) Anterior choroidal artery—arises from the posterior surface of the ICA 2 to 4 mm distal to the PCOM. It courses inferior and lateral to the optic tract in the suprasellar space as the **cisternal segment**, turns posteromedially around the uncus, and then posterolaterally through the **crural and ambient cisterns** to enter the **choroidal fissure** (plexal point) where the **plexal segment** in the temporal horn starts.

(i)   Cisternal segment—has 3 to 10 **perforators that supply the inferior optic chiasm, posterior $\frac{2}{3}$ of the optic tract, globus pallidus medius (GPm), genu of the internal capsule (IC), middle $\frac{1}{3}$ of the cerebral peduncle, substantia nigra (SN), upper red nucleus, subthalamus, and lateral parts of the ventral anterior (VA) and ventro lateral (VL) thalamic nuclei.**

(ii) Main artery—continues on to **supply the lateral $\frac{1}{2}$ of the geniculate body, inferior $\frac{1}{2}$ of the posterior limb of the IC, the retrolenticular IC, optic radiations, and choroid plexus of the lateral ventricles (along with the lateral posterior choroidal artery)**. It anastomoses with the lateral posterior choroidal arteries.

(iii) Aneurysms—tend to be located superior or superolaterally to the origin of the anterior choroidal artery.

(e) Dural artery—a small branch that arises from the ICA 3 to 5 mm proximal to the bifurcation and courses anteriorly to supply the dura of the anterior clinoid process.

(f) Carotid siphon—intracavernous and supraclinoid segments of the ICA.

G. Anterior cerebral artery (ACA) (**Fig. A–7**)

1. Twenty-five percent of the population have anomalies of the ACA (i.e., azygous), and these cases are more likely to be associated with aneurysms.

2. Precommunicating segment (A1)—has approximately eight perforators called the medial lenticulostriate arteries that **supply the superior surface of the optic nerve, optic chiasm, anterior hypothalamus, septum pellucidum, anterior commissure, pillars of fornix, and the anteroinferior striatum.** These perforators are also called the medial proximal striate arteries. The recurrent artery of Heubner is the medial distal striate artery.

3. Anterior communicating artery (ACOM)—located in the cistern of the lamina terminalis. Two or more perforators arise from the ACOM that **supply the infundibulum, optic chiasm, subcallosal area, and preoptic hypothalamus.** Perforators include the subcallosal artery and the medial artery of the corpus callosum. Aneurysms usually arise at the point where the dominant A1 bifurcates at the ACOM and points toward the opposite side.

4. Proximal pericallosal segment (A2)

   (a) **Recurrent artery of Heubner** (medial distal striate artery)—arises just proximal or **distal (most commonly) to the ACOM** and courses back toward the proximal A1, hence the term *recurrent*. It enters the **anterior perforating substance** and **supplies the head of the caudate, the anterior limb of the IC, the anterior putamen and globus pallidus (GP), the septal nuclei, and the inferior frontal lobe**.

   (b) Orbitofrontal artery (OFA)—supplies the gyrus rectus, medial orbital gyri, and the olfactory bulb and tract.

   (c) Frontopolar artery (FPA)—supplies the medial frontal lobe and lateral surface of the superior frontal gyrus.

   (d) Anterior internal frontal artery (AIFA)—supplies the anterior medial frontal lobe.

5. Segment distal to the pericallosal-callomarginal junction (A3)—generally **supplies the anterior $\frac{2}{3}$ of the medial cortex**.

   (a) Callosomarginal artery (CMA)—supplies the cingulate gyrus and paracentral lobule. It is the second most common aneurysm site on the ACA at the junction of the pericallosal artery, and the aneurysm usually points distally.

   (b) Pericallosal artery (PeCalA)—supplies the medial parietal cortex and the precuneus.

   (c) Middle internal frontal artery (MIFA)—supplies the medial frontal cortex.

   (d) Posterior internal frontal artery (PIFA)—supplies the medial posterior frontal cortex.

   (e) Paracentral artery (PceA)—supplies the medial cortex around the central sulcus.

   (f) Superior parietal artery (SPA)—supplies the medial superior parietal lobe.

   (g) Inferior parietal artery (IPA)—supplies the medial inferior parietal lobe.

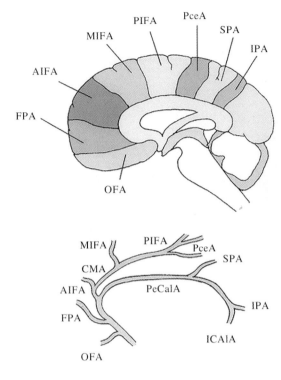

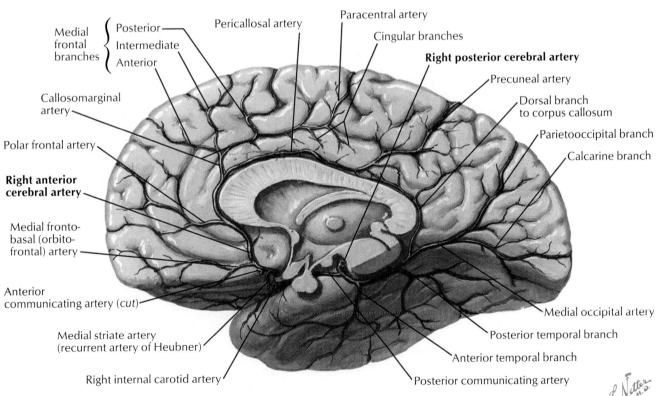

Note: Anterior parietal (postcentral sulcal) artery also occurs as separate anterior parietal and postcentral sulcal arteries

© Novartis

Figure A–7 *Anterior cerebral arteries (top) and anterior and posterior cerebral artery branches (bottom). IPA (inferior parietal artery), SPA (superior parietal artery), PceA (paracentral artery), PIFA (posterior internal frontal artery), MIFA (middle internal frontal artery), AIFA (anterior internal frontal artery), FPA (frontopolar artery), OFA (orbitofrontal artery), ICalA (inferior callosal artery), PeCalA (pericallosal artery), CMA (callosomarginal artery).*

H. Middle cerebral artery (MCA) (**Fig. A–8**)

1. **Sylvian point**—the most posterior branch of the MCA leaving the sylvian fissure, and it should be 5 cm from midline on an AP film.

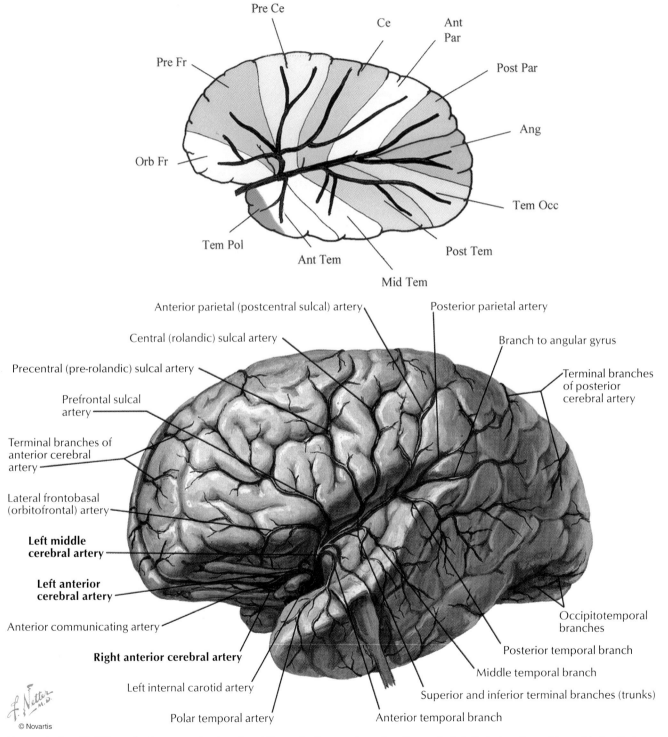

Figure A–8   Middle cerebral arteries (top) and middle cerebral artery branches (bottom). Orb Fr (orbitofrontal branch), Pre Fr (prefrontal branch), Pre Ce (precentral branch), Ce (central branch), Ant Par (anterior parietal branch), Post Par (posterior parietal branch), Ang (angular branch), Tem Occ (temporo-occipital branch), Post Tem (posterior temporal branch), Mid Tem (middle temporal branch), Ant Tem (anterior temporal branch), Tem Pol (temporopolar branch).

2. M1 segment (proximal to the bifurcation).

    (a) Uncal artery—more commonly arises from the distal ICA than the proximal M1 and supplies the uncus and underlying white matter.

    (b) Temporopolar artery (Tem Pol)—supplies the anterior pole of the superior, middle, and inferior temporal gyri.

    (c) Anterior temporal artery (Ant Tem)—supplies the anterior portion of the superior, middle, and inferior temporal gyri.

    (d) **Lateral lenticulostriate arteries**—2 to 15 perforators on the inferomedial surface of M1 that **supply the substantia innominata, lateral portion of the anterior commissure, most of the putamen, lateral segment of the GP, superior half of the IC, and the head and body of the caudate (except the anteroinferior portion)**.

3. M2 segment (from the bifurcation to the opercular branches leaving the sylvian fissure)

    (a) Superior trunk

        (i)   Orbitofrontal branch (Orb Fr)—supplies the orbital portion of the middle and inferior frontal gyri and the inferior pars orbitalis.

        (ii) Prefrontal branch (Pre Fr)—supplies the superior pars orbitalis, pars triangularis, anterior pars opercularis, and most of the middle frontal gyrus.

        (iii) Precentral branch (Pre Ce)—supplies the posterior pars opercularis, middle frontal gyrus, and inferior and middle portions of the precentral gyrus.

        (iv) Central branch (Ce)—supplies the superior postcentral gyrus, upper central sulcus, anterior part of the inferior parietal lobule, and the anteroinferior region of the superior parietal lobule.

        (v)   Anterior parietal branch (Ant Par)—supplies the superior parietal lobule.

    (b) Inferior trunk

        (i)   Posterior parietal (Post Par) branch—supplies the posterosuperior and inferior parietal lobule and the inferior supramarginal gyrus.

        (ii) Angular branch (Ang)—supplies the posterior aspect of the superior temporal gyrus, portions of the supramarginal and angular gyri, and the superior aspect of the lateral occipital gyrus.

        (iii) Temporo-occipital branch (Tem Occ)—supplies the posterior half of the superior temporal gyrus, posterior extreme of the middle and inferior temporal gyri, and the inferior lateral occipital gyrus.

        (iv) Posterotemporal branch (Post Tem)—supplies the middle and posterior parts of the superior temporal gyrus, posterior third of the middle temporal gyrus, and the posterior extreme of the inferior temporal gyrus.

        (v)   Middle temporal branch (Mid Tem)—supplies the superior temporal gyrus near the level of the pars triangularis and pars opercularis, central part of the middle temporal gyrus, and the middle and posterior parts of the inferior temporal gyrus.

4. The M3 segment (opercular branches emerging from the sylvian fissure)—a continuation of the M2 branches.

I.   Posterior cerebral artery (PCA) (**Fig. A–9**)

   1.   PCA—supplies the inferior temporal gyrus, occipital lobe, superior parietal lobule, brain stem, and the choroid of the third and lateral ventricles

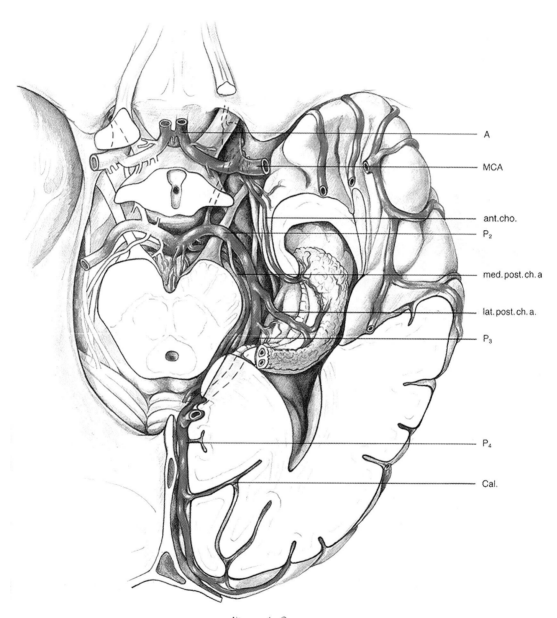

Figure A—9

Schematic drawing of the Circle of Willis and parapeduncular and peripheral course of the posterior cerebral artery (P_2, P_3, P_4) and its branches.

A	=	Anterior communicating artery complex
MCA	=	Middle cerebral artery
ant. cho.	=	anterior choroidal artery
P_2	=	P_2 segment
med. post. ch. a.	=	medial posterior choroidal artery
lat. post. ch. a.	=	lateral posterior choroidal artery
P_3	=	P_3 segment
P_4	=	P_4 segment
Cal.	=	Calcarine artery

2. P1 segment (in the peduncular cistern, proximal to PCOM junction)

   (a) Posterior thalamoperforator arteries—**supply the thalamus and midbrain**.

   (b) Medial posterior choroidal arteries—travel anteromedially along the roof of the third ventricle to **supply the midbrain tectum, posterior thalamus, pineal gland, and tela choroidea of the third ventricle**.

3. P2 segment (in the ambient cistern, extends from the PCOM junction to posterior to the quadrigeminal plate, travels around the midbrain and above the trochlear nerve and tentorial incisura)

   (a) Lateral posterior choroidal artery—**supplies the thalamus and the lateral ventricular choroid plexus**.

   (b) Medial and lateral thalamogeniculate arteries—**supply the medial geniculate bodies (MGBs), lateral geniculate bodies (LGBs), pulvinars, superior colliculis, and crus cerebri**.

4. P3 segment (in the quadrageminal cistern, begins posterior to the midbrain).

   (a) **Posterior temporal artery**—supplies the posterior temporal lobe, and the occipitotemporal and lingual gyri. It also has anterior temporal artery branches to the inferior temporal lobe that supply the inferior cortex and **anastomose with the MCA**.

   (b) **Internal occipital artery**

      (1) **Parieto-occipital artery**—supplies the posterior $\frac{1}{3}$ of the medial hemispheres and **anastomoses with the ACA**.

      (2) **Calcarine artery**—supplies the occipital pole and **anastomoses with the MCA**.

      (3) **Posterior pericallosal artery**—supplies the splenium of the corpus callosum and **anastomoses with the ACA**.

J. Anteromedial arteries—arise from the ACA and ACOM and enter the anterior perforated substance to supply the anterior hypothalamus, the preoptic nucleus, and the supraoptic nucleus.

K. Posteromedial arteries—arise from the PCOM and proximal PCA and supply the hypophysis, infundibulum, and tuberal hypothalamus. Thalamoperforating arteries supply the mamillary bodies, subthalamus, and midbrain.

L. Posterolateral arteries—arise from the PCA and supply the caudal thalamus (geniculate bodies, pulvinar, lateral nucleus, and lateral ventral nucleus) by way of the thalamogeniculate arteries.

M. Anterolateral arteries—the striate arteries from the proximal MCA and the recurrent artery of Heubner from the ACA that enter the anterior perforated substance to supply the striatum and the IC.

N. **Choroidal arteries**

1. Anterior choroidal artery—from the ICA and goes through the choroidal fissure to the temporal horn of the lateral ventricle to supply the choroid of the lateral ventricles, hippocampus, GP, posterior limb and retrolenticular IC, optic tract, amygdala, caudate tail, putamen, and ventral lateral (VL) thalamus. This artery had previously been sacrificed as a treatment for **Parkinson's disease** and tremor was decreased probably by decreasing the VL thalamus blood supply.

2. Posterior choroidal arteries—from the PCA and include medial branches that supply the pineal gland, tectum, choroid of the third ventricle, and thalamus, and lateral branches that enter the choroidal fissure and anastomose with the anterior choroidal arteries to form a variable anastomotic network.

O. Striatum—supplied mainly by the **MCA by way of the lenticulostriate arteries**, rostrally by the **recurrent artery of Heubner**, and caudally by the **anterior choroidal artery**.

P. **Lateral internal capsule**—supplied by the MCA by way of lenticulostriate branches, the anterior limb by the recurrent artery of Heubner, the genu by the ICA perforators, and the posterior limb by the anterior choroidal artery and PCOM artery.

Q. **Thalamus**—supplied by the **PCA** by way of posterior thalamoperforators, thalamogeniculate arteries, and the medial posterior choroidal arteries. It also receives supply rostrally from the **PCOM (anterior thalamoperforating arteries)** and the basilar bifurcation perforators (posterior thalamoperforating arteries).

R. Ventricular supply—the **lateral ventricles are supplied by the anterior choroidal and lateral posterior choroidal arteries**. The **third ventricle is supplied by the medial posterior choroidal arteries**. The **fourth ventricle is supplied by the SCA, AICA, and PICA**. The AICA passes adjacent to the foramen of Luschka.

S. Circle of Willis—consists of the anterior communicating artery (ACOM) connecting both right and left anterior cerebral arteries and the posterior communicating arteries (PCOM) connecting the internal carotid arteries with the posterior cerebral arteries (from the basilar artery trunk). The Circle of Willis allows blood from any of the 4 major brain supply vessels (bilateral internal carotid arteries and vertebral arteries) to circle around to a deficiently perfused area. It is complete in 25% of individuals. 50% have posterior circulation variations (hypoplasia, etc.). **(Figs. A–10 and A–11)**

T. Supratentorial venous drainage **(Figs. A–12—A–14)**

1. Cerebral veins—have no valves.

2. Emissary veins—go from the scalp to the dural sinuses or vice versa.

3. Superior sagittal sinus—extends from the foramen cecum to the torcula and usually drains predominantly into the **right transverse sinus**.

4. Inferior sagittal sinus—joins the vein of Galen and drains into the straight sinus that drains into the torcula and usually predominantly into the **left transverse sinus**.

5. Cavernous sinus—connected by a basilar venous plexus an each side both anterior and posterior to the hypophysis. It drains into the **superior petrosal sinus to the transverse/sigmoid sinus junction** and the **inferior petrosal sinus to the jugular bulb**. It is also connected to the pterygoid and pharyngeal venous plexuses.

6. Superficial veins **(Fig. A–15)**

(a) Superior cerebral vein (vein of Trolard)—drains from the sylvian fissure into the superior sagittal sinus.

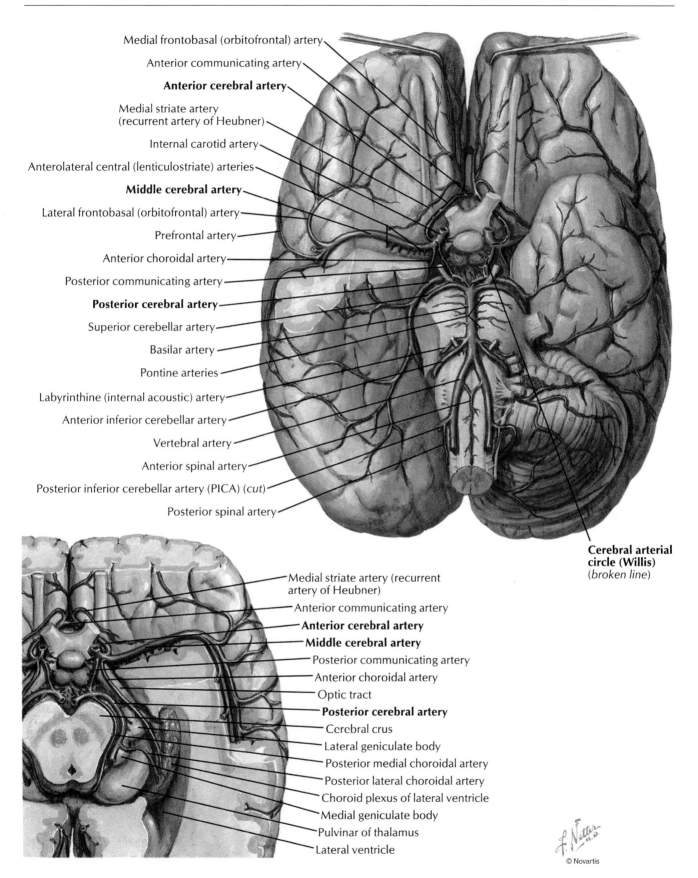

Medial frontobasal (orbitofrontal) artery

Anterior communicating artery

Anterior cerebral artery

Medial striate artery
(recurrent artery of Heubner)

Internal carotid artery

Anterolateral central (lenticulostriate) arteries

Middle cerebral artery

Lateral frontobasal (orbitofrontal) artery

Prefrontal artery

Anterior choroidal artery

Posterior communicating artery

Posterior cerebral artery

Superior cerebellar artery

Basilar artery

Pontine arteries

Labyrinthine (internal acoustic) artery

Anterior inferior cerebellar artery

Vertebral artery

Anterior spinal artery

Posterior inferior cerebellar artery (PICA) (*cut*)

Posterior spinal artery

**Cerebral arterial
circle (Willis)**
(*broken line*)

Medial striate artery (recurrent
artery of Heubner)

Anterior communicating artery

Anterior cerebral artery

Middle cerebral artery

Posterior communicating artery

Anterior choroidal artery

Optic tract

Posterior cerebral artery

Cerebral crus

Lateral geniculate body

Posterior medial choroidal artery

Posterior lateral choroidal artery

Choroid plexus of lateral ventricle

Medial geniculate body

Pulvinar of thalamus

Lateral ventricle

Figure A–10   Circle of Willis and branches (top) and axial slice of circle of Willis.

Vessels dissected out: inferior view

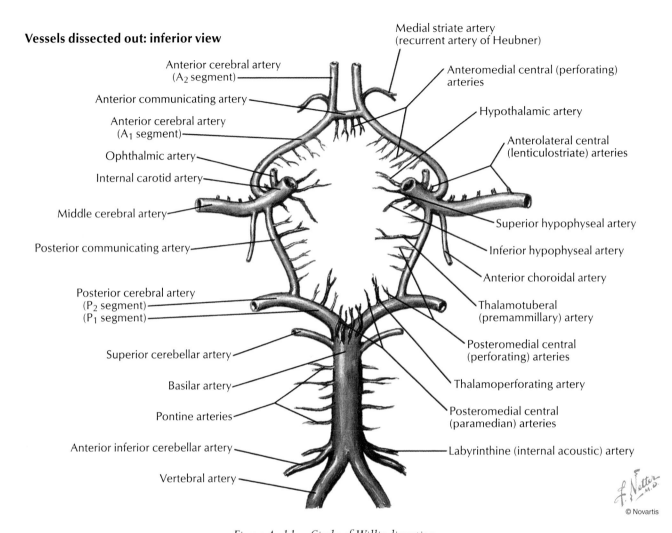

Figure A–11   *Circle of Willis dissection.*

Figure A–12   *Venous anatomy.*

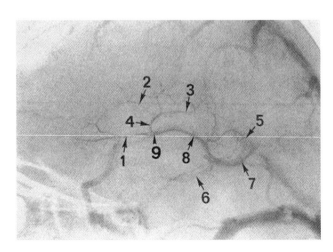

1 Septal vein
2 Anterior caudate vein
3 Terminal vein
4 Thalamostriate vein
5 Atrial vein
6 Basal vein of Rosenthal
7 Vein of Galen
8 Internal cerebral vein
9 Venous angle

Sagittal section

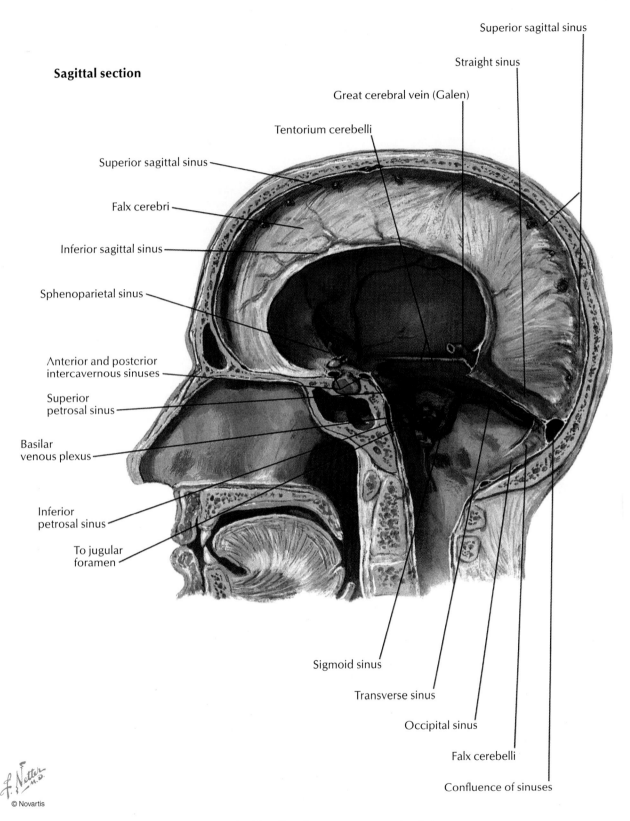

Superior sagittal sinus

Straight sinus

Great cerebral vein (Galen)

Tentorium cerebelli

Superior sagittal sinus

Falx cerebri

Inferior sagittal sinus

Sphenoparietal sinus

Anterior and posterior intercavernous sinuses

Superior petrosal sinus

Basilar venous plexus

Inferior petrosal sinus

To jugular foramen

Sigmoid sinus

Transverse sinus

Occipital sinus

Falx cerebelli

Confluence of sinuses

© Novartis

Figure A–13   Dural venous sinuses, sagittal view.

**Skull sectioned horizontally:
superior view**

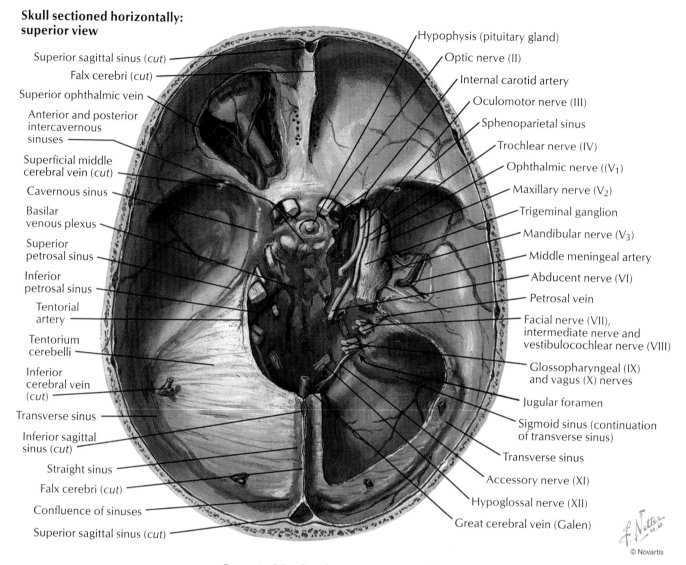

Superior sagittal sinus (*cut*)

Falx cerebri (*cut*)

Superior ophthalmic vein

Anterior and posterior
intercavernous
sinuses

Superficial middle
cerebral vein (*cut*)

Cavernous sinus

Basilar
venous plexus

Superior
petrosal sinus

Inferior
petrosal sinus

Tentorial
artery

Tentorium
cerebelli

Inferior
cerebral vein
(*cut*)

Transverse sinus

Inferior sagittal
sinus (*cut*)

Straight sinus

Falx cerebri (*cut*)

Confluence of sinuses

Superior sagittal sinus (*cut*)

Hypophysis (pituitary gland)

Optic nerve (II)

Internal carotid artery

Oculomotor nerve (III)

Sphenoparietal sinus

Trochlear nerve (IV)

Ophthalmic nerve ((V₁)

Maxillary nerve (V₂)

Trigeminal ganglion

Mandibular nerve (V₃)

Middle meningeal artery

Abducent nerve (VI)

Petrosal vein

Facial nerve (VII),
intermediate nerve and
vestibulocochlear nerve (VIII)

Glossopharyngeal (IX)
and vagus (X) nerves

Jugular foramen

Sigmoid sinus (continuation
of transverse sinus)

Transverse sinus

Accessory nerve (XI)

Hypoglossal nerve (XII)

Great cerebral vein (Galen)

© Novartis

Figure A–14   Dural venous sinuses, axial view.

(b) Inferior cerebral veins—drain into the basal sinuses (cavernous, petrosal, and transverse).

(c) Superficial middle cerebral veins (in the sylvian fissure)—drain to the cavernous sinus, the vein of Trolard, and to the vein of Labbé.

(d) **Vein of Labbé**—drains from the sylvian fissure into the **transverse sinus**.

7. Deep veins—drain deep white matter and subcortical structures.

(a) **Internal cerebral veins**—located in the tela choroidea of the roof of the third ventricle (velum interpositum) that extends from the interventricular foramen, travel over the thalamus and posteriorly to the quadragerminal cistern, where they join to contribute to the vein of Galen. They are formed by the **union of the thalamostriate, choroidal, septal, epithalamic, and lateral ventricular veins**.

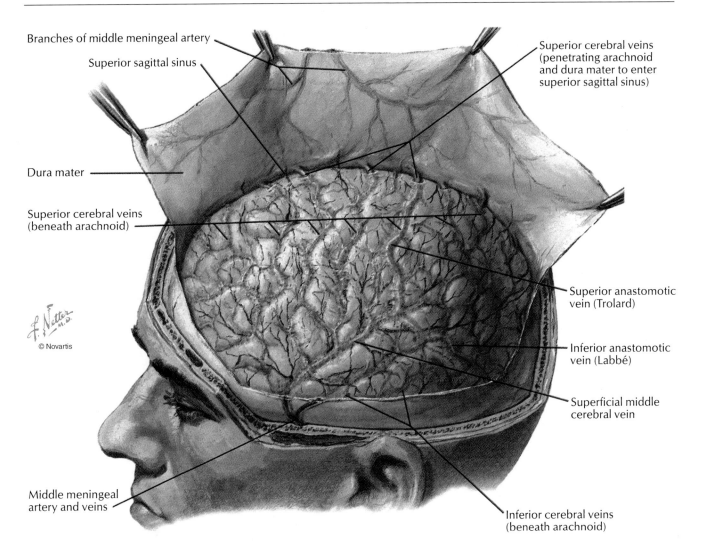

Branches of middle meningeal artery

Superior sagittal sinus

Dura mater

Superior cerebral veins
(beneath arachnoid)

Middle meningeal
artery and veins

Superior cerebral veins
(penetrating arachnoid
and dura mater to enter
superior sagittal sinus)

Superior anastomotic
vein (Trolard)

Inferior anastomotic
vein (Labbé)

Superficial middle
cerebral vein

Inferior cerebral veins
(beneath arachnoid)

Figure A–15   Superficial cerebral veins.

(b) **Basal vein of Rosenthal**—drains the **anterior and medial temporal lobe**, passes posterosuperiorly through the **ambient cistern**, and joins the internal cerebral vein to form the vein of Galen.

(c) **Vein of Galen**—receives both internal cerebral veins, both basal veins of Rosenthal, the occipital veins, and a posterior callosal vein. It travels under the splenium and merges with the inferior sagittal sinus to form the straight sinus.

U. Vertebral artery and branches

1. Vertebral artery—arises from the subclavian artery, enters the foramina transversarium at C6, turns laterally at C2, travels posteriorly along the atlas, and then enters the skull through the foramen magnum. The left side is dominant 50%, right side dominant 25%, and no dominance

25%. Forty percent of people have one hypoplastic vertebral artery. The left vertebral artery arises from the aorta in 5% of cases. Multiple anastomoses exist with the ECA, thyrocervical trunk, and costocervical trunk. It supplies the pyramids, the inferior olivary nucleus, the vagal and hypoglossal nuclei, and the reticular formation.

2. Posterior spinal artery—supplies the gracile and cuneate fasciculi and the inferior cerebellar peduncle.

3. Anterior spinal artery—supplies the pyramid, medial lemniscus (ML), medial longitudinal fasciculus (MLF), olive, and the vagal and hypoglossal nuclei.

4. Posterior inferior cerebellar artery (PICA)—occasionally arises extracranially. One to 25% of vertebral arteries terminate in a PICA. It has an anterior medullary segment, lateral medullary segment (supplies CNs IX, X, and to XI), tonsillomedullary segment, and telovelotonsilar (between the tela choroidea and inferior medullary velum rostrally and the tonsils caudally) segments. It supplies the choroid of the fourth ventricle, posterior lateral medulla, tonsils, vermis, and posteroinferior hemispheres. Occlusion causes **Wallenberg's** or **lateral medullary syndrome** (also may be due to vertebral artery occlusion), with ipsilateral loss of pain and temperature sensation on the face and contralateral loss on the body, ipsilateral weakness of the pharynx and larynx, ipsilateral cerebellar limb ataxia, and ipsilateral Horner's syndrome.

5. Posterior meningeal artery—arises near the atlas and supplies the falx cerebelli (also supplied by the occipital, ascending pharyngeal, and PICA arteries).

V. Basilar artery branches

1. Anterior inferior cerebellar artery (AICA)—crosses the abducens nerve and the cerebellopontine angle (CPA) cistern to the internal auditory canal and passes anterior and inferior to CN VII and VIII. It supplies CN VII, VIII, the inferior lateral pons, middle cerebellar peduncle, flocculus, and the anterolateral hemispheres. Branches include the internal auditory artery, recurrent perforating artery, and subarcuate artery.

2. Labyrinthine artery—supplies the structures of the labyrinth.

3. Paramedian artery—supplies the ventral pons and midbrain.

4. Long and short circumferential pontine arteries—supply the ventral pons.

5. Superior cerebellar artery (SCA)—travels below CN III and IV to supply the superior vermis and cerebellar hemispheres, deep white matter, and **deep nuclei**.

6. Posterior cerebellar arteries (PCA)–discussed above.

W. Pons—supplied by the basilar paramedian branches and the short and long circumferential branches that anastomose with AICA at the middle cerebellar peduncle.

X.   Midbrain—supplied by the basilar artery, PCA, SCA, PCOM, and anterior choroidal artery. Stroke syndromes include (1) **Weber's syndrome** with ipsilateral oculomotor weakness and contralateral hemiplegia, and (2) **Benedikt's syndrome**, an infarction of the red nucleus, superior cerebellar peduncle, and oculomotor nucleus.

Y.   Cerebellum—supplied by (1) PICA to the inferior cerebellar peduncle, vermis, tonsils, and the choroid of the fourth ventricle; (2) AICA to the middle cerebellar peduncle, choroid of the fourth ventricle, and the anterior cerebellum; and (3) SCA to the superior cerebellar peduncle, the choroid of the fourth ventricle, and the **deep nuclei**.

Z.   Venous drainage—by way of the superior median (precentral cerebellar) vein to the vein of Galen, the inferior median vein to the straight and transverse sinuses, and the superior and lateral veins to the superior and inferior petrosal sinuses.

V. BLOOD SUPPLY TO THE SPINAL CORD

A.   Paired posterior spinal arteries—lie medial to the dorsal roots and supply the **posterior $\frac{1}{3}$ of the spinal cord**.

B.   Two anterior spinal arteries—join at the medulla and enter the anterior median fissure as the anterior median spinal artery to supply the **anterior $\frac{2}{3}$** of the full length of the spinal cord. Anterior radicular arteries anastomose with this system.

C.   Anterior and posterior spinal arteries—supply most of the cervical cord.

D.   Distal cord—supplied by radicular anastamoses that enter through the intervertebral foramen and divide into anterior and posterior radicular arteries which are more prominent on the left side and join the spinal artery system.

E.   Upper region (C1-T3)

    1.   C1-4—supplied by the anterior and posterior spinal arteries.

    2.   C5-6—supplied by ascending vertebral artery branches and the thyrocervical trunk.

    3.   C7-T3—supplied by the costocervical trunk.

F.   Middle region (T4-8)—the **most vulnerable to low flow** and supplied mainly by a single thoracic radicular artery at T7 from the aorta.

G.   Lower region (T9-sacrum)—supplied mainly by the single **left** T11 great radicular **artery of Adamkiewicz** (75% from T10-12). The aorta and iliac arteries sends branches to the thoracolumbar spine. The lateral sacral artery supplies the sacral neural elements.

H.   Posterior system—supplies smaller but more evenly distributed posterior radicular arteries. It forms a leptomeningeal perimedullary network that anastomoses with the anterior system, most prominently at the level of the conus where the anastomotic loop is located. The blood from posterior medullary arteries flows *centripetally* in the perforating branches from the leptomeningeal system from the spinal cord surface to the posterior columns and posterior horns.

I. Anterior system—feeds into the anterior medullary artery in the anterior median fissure and flows *centrifugally* by way of penetrating branches to the anterior and intermediate gray and by way of a pial radial network to the white matter of the anterior and lateral funiculi.

J. There are 2 to 17 anterior radicular arteries; usually <6 cervical arteries, 2 to 4 thoracic arteries, and 1 to 2 lumbar arteries. The artery of Adamkiewicz enters at the lower thoracic or upper lumbar spine.

K. There are 10 to 23 posterior radicular arteries.

L. The anterior ramus of the segmental artery supplies the cord (usually small branches but larger at T4-9) and the posterior ramus branches in the foramen to supply the dorsal root ganglion (DRG) and nerve roots by way of the anterior and posterior radicular branches.

M. Most vulnerable areas of the spinal cord—at T1-4 and L1. An intercostal artery occlusion or an aortic dissection may cause a cord stroke here. A watershed area also exists between the anterior and posterior medullary arteries' territories between the intermediate and dorsal horns and lateral and posterior fasciculi.

N. Venous drainage—variable. An anterior median spinal vein and two posterior coronal veins drain rostrally up to the head.

VI. INTRACRANIAL-EXTRACRANIAL ANASTOMOSES

A. Ascending pharyngeal artery to vertebral artery at C3 and to the ICA's petrous and cavernous branches.

B. Facial artery's angular branch to the ICA by way of the orbital to ophthalmic branches.

C. Occipital artery to vertebral artery at C1 and C2.

D. Posterior auricular artery to the ICA by way of the stylomastoid artery.

E. Maxillary artery to ICA.

    1. Middle meningeal artery to the ethmoidal branch of ophthalmic artery.

    2. Artery of the foramen rotundum to the inferior lateral trunk of the ICA.

    3. Accessory meningeal artery to the inferior lateral trunk of the ICA.

    4. Vidian artery to the infratemporal ICA.

    5. Anterior and deep temporal arteries to the ophthalmic artery by way of lacrimal, palpebral, and muscular branches.

VII. PERSISTENT FETAL CAROTID-VERTEBRAL ANASTOMOSES (FIG. A–16)

A. **Primitive trigeminal artery**—the most frequent of the persistent fetal circulations (besides fetal PCOM) and is present in 0.1 to 0.5% of people. The vessel arises from the ICA just proximal to the cavernous sinus or just proximal to the meningohypophyseal trunk and curves medially to join the basilar artery between the SCA and AICA. It is associated with increased frequency of aneurysms and arterio-venus malformations (AVMs) (as are the other types of persistent fetal circulations) (**Fig. A–17**).

B. Persistent otic/acoustic artery—connects the petrous ICA through the internal auditory meatus to the basilar artery.

C. Primitive hypoglossal artery—the second most frequent, it occurs in 0.1% of cases. The vessel arises from the cervical ICA and connects to the basilar artery through the hypoglossal canal.

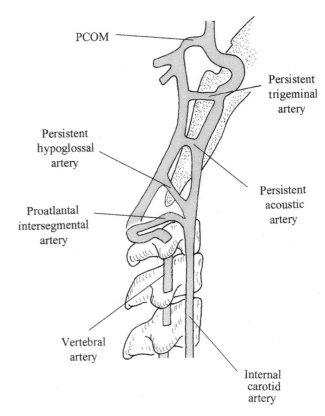

Figure A–16   Persistent fetal circulation.

D. Proatlantal intersegmental artery—a suboccipital anastamoses between the ECA or cervical ICA to the vertebral artery between the arch of C1 and the occiput.

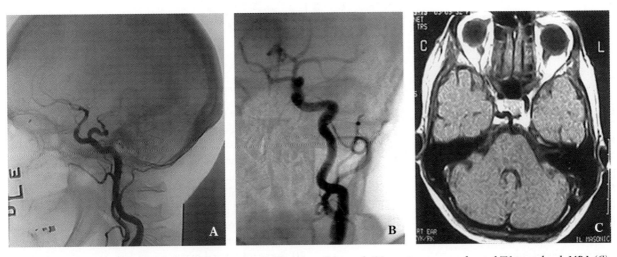

Figure A–17   Persistent trigeminal artery (angiogram). AP (A) and lateral (B) angiograms and axial T1-weighted MRI (C) with flow void of primitive artery.

VIII. CORTICAL ANATOMY

A. General anatomy (**Figs. A–18—A–21**)

    1. The cortex has 14 billion neurons.

    2. Cells that develop later pass more superficially from the germinal zone and form connections with the cells they pass.

    3. Cell types —pyramidal (main output), stellate, and fusiform.

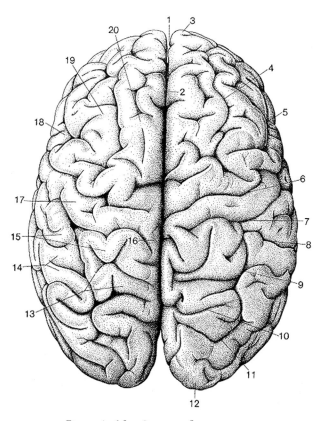

Figure A–18   Brain surface anatomy.

  1 Longitudinal fissure of cerebrum
  2 Superior margin of cerebrum
  3 Frontal pole
  4 Superior frontal sulcus
  5 Inferior frontal sulcus
  6 Precentral sulcus
  7 Central sulcus
  8 Postcentral sulcus
  9 Intraparietal sulcus
10 Parieto-occipital sulcus

11 Transverse occipital sulcus
12 Occipital pole
13 Superior parietal lobule
14 Inferior parietal lobule
15 Postcentral gyrus
16 Paracentral lobule
17 Precentral gyrus
18 Inferior frontal gyrus
19 Middle frontal gyrus
20 Superior frontal gyrus

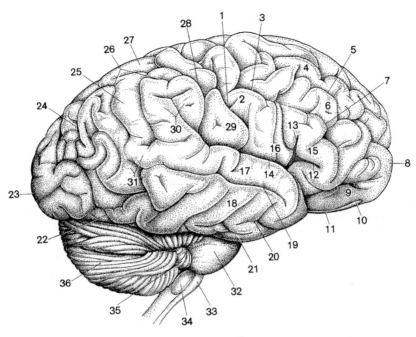

Figure A–19 Brain surface anatomy.

1 Central sulcus
2 Precentral gyrus
3 Precentral sulcus
4 Superior frontal gyrus
5 Superior frontal sulcus
6 Middle frontal gyrus
7 Inferior frontal sulcus
8 Frontal pole
9 Orbital gyri
10 Olfactory bulb
11 Olfactory tract
12–14 *Lateral sulcus* (in depth: lateral cerebral fossa)
12 Anterior ramus
13 Ascending ramus
14 Posterior ramus
15 Frontal operculum
16 Frontoparietal operculum
17 Superior temporal gyrus
18 Middle temporal gyrus

19 Superior temporal sulcus
20 Inferior temporal sulcus
21 Inferior temporal gyrus
22 Preoccipital notch
23 Occipital pole
24 Transverse occipital sulcus
25 Inferior parietal lobule
26 Intraparietal sulcus
27 Superior parietal lobule
28 Postcentral sulcus
29 Postcentral gyrus
30 Supramarginal gyrus
31 Angular gyrus
32 Pons
33 Pyramid (medulla oblongata)
34 Olive
35 Flocculus
36 Cerebellar hemisphere

4. Neurotransmitters—glutamate and aspartate (excitatory), and GABA (inhibitory, stays in the cortex, and augmented by barbiturates and anticonvulsants).

5. Isocortex or neocortex—has six layers.

6. **Allocortex—has three layers** and is found in the olfactory cortex, hippocampus, and dentate gyrus.

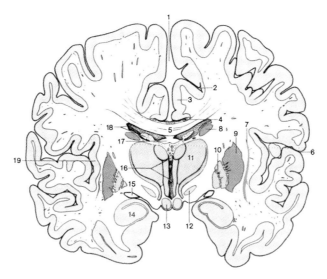

Figure A–20   Brain surface anatomy.

1 Longitudinal fissure of cerebrum
2 Cingulate sulcus
3 Cingulate gyrus
4 Sulcus of corpus callosum
5 Corpus callosum
6 Lateral sulcus
7 Claustrum
8–9 *Corpus striatum*
8 Caudate nucleus
9 Putamen
9, 10 *Lentiform nucleus*

10 *Globus pallidus*
11 Thalamus
12 Subthalamic nucleus
13 Mamillary body
14 Amygdaloid body
15 Optic tract
16 3rd ventricle and its choroid plexus
17 Body of fornix
18 Lateral ventricle and its choroid plexus
19 Cortex of insula

B. Layers (**Fig. A–22**)

1. Molecular layer—the most superficial and contains horizontal axons and Golgi 2 cells.

2. External granular layer—contains granule cells.

3. External pyramidal layer—involved with commisural fibers.

4. Internal granular layer—contains stellate cells and the external band of Baillarger.

5. Internal pyramidal layer—contains the largest cells.

6. Multiform layer.

7. Fiber types—the projection fibers are in specific descending tracts, association fibers connect cortex to cortex, and commisural fibers connect cortex to the contralateral side.

8. **Layers 1 and 2**—receive diffuse afferent fibers from the lower brain to control the excitability of the region.

9. **Layer 3** fibers—connect the two hemispheres. Layers 2 and 3 also have ipsilateral corticocortico association fibers.

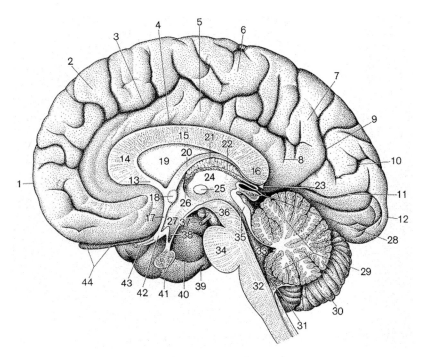

Figure A–21   Brain surface anatomy.

1 Frontal lobe: frontal pole
2 Medial frontal gyrus
3 Cingulate sulcus
4 Sulcus of corpus callosum
5 Cingulate gyrus
6 Paracentral lobule
7 Precuneus
8 Subparietal sulcus
9 Parieto-occipital sulcus
10 Cuneus
11 Calcarine fissure
12 Occipital lobe: occipital pole
13–16 *Corpus callosum* (cut surface)
13 Rostrum
14 Genu
15 Trunk
16 Splenium
17 Lamina terminalis (cut surface)
18 Anterior commissure (cut surface)
19 Septum pellucidum
20 Fornix
21 Tela choroidea of 3rd ventricle
22 Choroid plexus of 3rd ventricle (cut edge)

23 Transverse cerebral fissure
24 Thalamus
25 Interthalamic adhesion (cut surface)
26 Interventricular foramen
27 Hypothalamus
28 Suprapineal recess and pineal body (cut surface)
29 Vermis of cerebellum (cut surface)
30 Cerebellar hemisphere
31 Choroid plexus of 4th ventricle
32 Medulla oblongata (cut surface)
33 4th ventricle
34 Pons (cut surface)
35 Tectal lamina (cut surface) and mesencephalic aqueduct
36 Mamillary body
37 Oculomotor nerve
38 Infundibular recess
39 Temporal lobe: lateral occipitotemporal gyrus
40 Rhinal fissure
41 Hypophysis (cut surface) with adenohypophysis (anterior) and neurohypophysis
42 Optic chiasma (cut surface)
43 Optic nerve
44 Olfactory bulb and tract

10. **Layer 4**—the main sensory afferent input and is enlarged in sensory cortex.

11. **Layer 5**—the main efferent supply to the brain stem and spinal cord and is enlarged in motor cortex.

12. **Layer 6**—contains efferent fibers to the thalamus.

C. Brodmann's areas (**Table A–1; Fig. A–23**)

D. Sensory cortices—the somesthetic area (areas 3, 1, 2), the visual area (area 17), the auditory area (areas 41, 42), the gustatory area (area 43), and the olfactory area (no distinct Brodmann number).

1. **Primary somesthetic area** (SI)—in the postcentral gyrus. Input is from the VPLc and the VPM thalamic nuclei that also project to the SII area. **Area 3a has input from muscle spindles, 3b from skin, 1 from either, and 2 from deep (joint) receptors.** The face and tongue have bilateral representation (**Fig. A–24**).

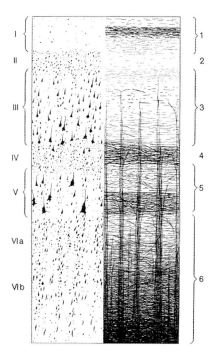

Figure A–22   Isocortex layers.

I–VI	Cell layers
I–III	External principal zone
IV–VI	Internal principal zone
1–6	Myelinated layers

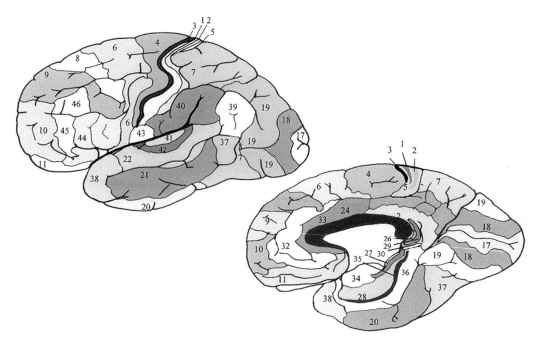

Figure A–23   Brodmann's areas.

TABLE A–1. BRODMANN'S AREAS

Brodmann's area	Functional area	Location	Function
1, 2, 3	Primary somatosensory cortex	Postcentral gyrus	Touch
4	Primary motor cortex	Precentral gyrus	Voluntary motor control
5	Tertiary somatosensory cortex; posterior parietal association area	Superior parietal lobule	Stereognosia
6	Supplementary motor control; supplementary eye field; premotor cortex; frontal eye fields	Precentral gyrus and rostral adjacent cortex	Limb and eye movement planning
7	Posterior parietal association area	Superior parietal lobule	Visuomotor; perception
8	Frontal eye fields	Superior, middle frontal gyri, medial frontal lobe	Saccadic eye movements
9, 10, 11, 12	Prefrontal association cortex; frontal eye fields	Superior, middle frontal gyri, medial frontal lobe	Thought, cognition, movement planning
13, 14, 15, 16		Insular cortex	
17	Primary visual cortex	Banks of calcarine fissure	Vision
18	Secondary visual cortex	Medial and lateral occipital gyri	Vision; depth
19	Tertiary visual cortex, middle temporal visual area	Medial and lateral occipital gyri	Vision, color, motion, depth
20	Visual inferotemporal area	Inferior temporal gyrus	Form vision
21	Visual inferotemporal area	Middle temporal gyrus	Form vision
22	Higher order auditory cortex	Superior temporal gyrus	Hearing, speech
23, 24, 25, 26, 27	Limbic association cortex	Cingulate gyrus, subcallosal area, retrosplenial area, parahippocampal gyrus	Emotions
28	Primary olfactory cortex; limbic association cortex	Parahippocampal gyrus	Smell, emotions
29, 30, 31, 32, 33	Limbic association cortex	Cingulate gyrus and retrosplenial area	Emotions
34, 35, 36	Primary olfactory cortex; limbic association cortex	Parahippocampal gyrus	Smell, emotions
37	Parietal-temporal-occipital association cortex; middle temporal visual area	Middle and inferior temporal gyri at temporo occipital junction	Perception, vision, reading, speech
38	Primary olfactory cortex; limbic association cortex	Temporal pole	Smell, emotions
39	Parietal-temporal-occipital association cortex	Inferior parietal lobule (angular gyrus)	Perception, vision, reading, speech
40	Parietal-temporal-occipital association cortex	Inferior parietal lobule (supramarginal gyrus)	Perception, vision, reading, speech

TABLE A–1 (CONTINUED). BRODMANN'S AREAS

Brodmann's area	Functional area	Location	Function
41	Primary auditory cortex	Heschl's gyri and superior temporal gyrus	Hearing
42	Secondary auditory cortex	Heschl's gyri and superior temporal gyrus	Hearing
43	Gustatory cortex	Insular cortex, fronto parietal operculum	Taste
44	Broca's area; lateral premotor cortex	Inferior frontal gyrus (frontal operculum)	Speech, movement planning
45	Prefrontal association cortex	Inferior frontal gyrus (frontal operculum)	Thought, cognition, planning behavior
46	Prefrontal association cortex (dorsolateral prefrontal cortex)	Middle frontal gyrus	Thought, cognition, planning behavior, eye movement
47	Prefrontal association cortex	Inferior frontal gyrus (frontal operculum)	Thought, cognition, planning behavior

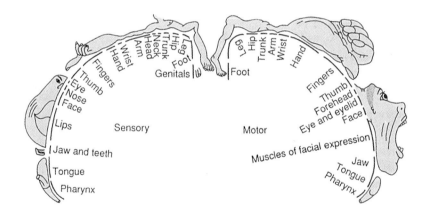

Figure A–24   Motor and sensory homunculus.

2. **Secondary somesthetic area** (SII)—on the superior bank of the lateral sulcus. Input is from the ipsilateral VPLc, VPM, and bilateral SI. Efferent fibers go to the ipsilateral SI and the motor cortex. Information is bilateral and the **homunculus is inverted with the face rostral**.

3. **Primary visual cortex** (area 17) or striate cortex—in the walls and floors of the calcarine sulcus. Input is from the geniculocalcarine fibers of the lateral geniculate body (LGB) to the external sagittal stratum. Output is from the internal sagittal stratum by way of corticofugal fibers to the superior colliculus and the LGB. The macula projects to the posterior $\frac{1}{3}$ of the calcarine cortex (occipital pole). The vertical meridian has commissural fibers for bilateral representation. The receptive field of a ganglion cell is the region of the retina that affects the firing of one retinal ganglion cell. It is either on-center and off-surround or off-center and

on-surround. These cells fire at a constant steady rate. The LGB also has on and off areas and contributes to visual processing. The cortex no longer has concentric receptive fields. The ocular dominance columns have alternating right and left stripes. Orientation columns each represent 180 degrees. The **band of Baillarger** in the striate cortex is the **stripe of Gennari** visible to the naked eye: the recognizable **layer IVb** on myelin-stained sections caused by the presence of a dense plexus of myelinated axons that are collaterals of the primary visual cortical axons.

4. **Secondary visual areas** V-II (area 18) and V-III (area 19, more lateral)—input from the LGB and pulvinar.

5. **Primary auditory cortex** (area 41)—the **two transverse gyri of Heschl** that are donsomedial (DM) to the superior temporal convolution and buried on the temporal operculum of the sylvian fissure. The association area is 42 and surrounds area 41. Input is from the MGB with fibers that pass through the sublenticular IC. The ventral MGB has tonotopic organization with high frequencies medial. The dorsal and medial MGB go to the ipsilateral area 41. Isofrequency cell columns are present in the cortex. **Each cochlea projects bilaterally but more to the contralateral side.** A unilateral lesion causes partial deafness bilaterally, but mainly contralaterally. **The trapezoid body is the only auditory commissure needed for sound localization.** A lesion in area 22 of the dominant hemisphere causes word deafness or sensory aphasia with normal hearing.

6. **Gustatory area** (area 43)—in the postcentral operculum adjacent to the tongue sensory area. Input is from the ipsilateral nucleus solitarius to the VPMpc to area 43.

7. **Vestibular cortex**—in area 3a and 2 of SI with bilateral representation, although more contralaterally.

E. Motor cortex

1. **Primary motor cortex** MI (area 4)—for voluntary motor control. The pyramidal cells of Betz make up **3%** of the corticospinal fibers. The corticospinal fibers are **31%** from area 4, **29%** from area 6, and **40%** from the parietal cortex. The main neurotransmitters are glutamate and aspartate (+). The corticospinal tract is **not somatotopic**. The corticospinal tract projects mainly unilaterally but is bilateral for eye, face, and tongue movements. Columns may be present as in the visual and somatosensory cortex.

2. **Premotor cortex** (area 6a)—controls voluntary motor responses dependent on sensory input. It is on the lateral aspect of the cortex anterior to area 4. A unilateral lesion produces no deficit.

3. **Supplemental motor cortex** MII (area 6a)—involved with the programming, planning, and initiating of motor movement. There is somatotopic organization of neurons. It is on the medial aspect of the hemisphere anterior to area 4 on the medial superior frontal gyrus and receives bilateral input. Output is to ipsilateral areas 4, 6, 5, and 7, contralateral MII, bilateral spinal cord, caudate, putamen, and thalamus. A lesion here causes akinesis and **diminished spontaneous speech**.

4. Input to the motor area—from the ipsilateral thalamic VL and VPLo and the contralateral cerebellum to MI; the mGP to the ipsilateral thalamic VApc, VLo, and CM to MII and premotor cortex but not MI; SI to all but not from area 3; and MII to MI and premotor cortex.

5. **Frontal eye fields** (area 8)—rostral to the premotor area in the caudal **middle frontal gyrus**. They initiate **saccades**. Stimulation causes contralateral eye deviation. A lesion causes impaired saccades, especially if in the dominant hemisphere. The occipital eye center (area 17) controls contralateral pursuit. **The eye fields do not reach the CN nuclei III, IV, and VI directly** but go to the rostral interstitial nucleus of the MLF, the interstitial nucleus of Cajal, the PPRF, and the superior colliculus.

6. The motor cortex has reciprocal fibers with the thalamus, except for the thalamic reticular nuclei that receive afferent fibers from the entire cortex but do not send them back. The prefrontal cortex sends fibers to the intralaminar thalamic nuclei.

F. Cerebral dominance

1. Cerebral dominance exists for language and handedness

    (a) Right-handed people—nearly always **left brain language dominant**.

    (b) Left-handed people—left hemispheric dominant 85%, bilaterally dominant 15%, and rarely right side dominant.

    (c) **Dominant hemisphere (usually left)—controls language, arithmetic, and analytical thought.**

    (d) **Nondominant hemisphere (usually right)—involved with spatial analysis, face recognition, music, and emotion**. Pictures may communicate language to the nondominant hemisphere, but letters need the dominant hemisphere for analysis. Sign language uses mainly the left hemisphere.

    (e) Men are more frequently left-handed, dyslexic, and stutterers. Handedness may be determined by testosterone during brain development.

2. Lesion in the nondominant inferior parietal lobule—causes neglect, a failure to recognize a side of the body.

3. Lesion in the dominant angular and supramarginal gyri—causes **Gerstmann's syndrome** with right/left dissociation, finger agnosia, acalculia, and agraphia.

4. Gnosis is memory. It is lost with sensory association damage. Aphasia is gnosis of language. Apraxia is the inability to perform a learned movement without lack of comprehension, weakness, or a sensory deficit.

IX. DIENCEPHALON

A. General information

1. The diencephalon contains the epithalamus, thalamus, hypothalamus, subthalamus, and metathalamus (MGB and LGB).

2. It extends from the posterior commissure to the foramen of Monro. The lateral border is the posterior limb of the IC, tail of the caudate, and stria terminalis.

3. The inferior aspect near the midbrain junction contains the pulvinar, MGB, LGB, and the retrolenticular IC.

4. The epithalamus contains the pineal gland, habenular trigones, stria medullaris, and roof of the third ventricle.

B. Habenulum

1. **Habenular nucleus** and commissure—involved with convergence of limbic pathways and have output into the midbrain.

2. Input—from the GP to the lateral habenulum and from the **stria medullaris** with fibers from the septal nuclei, lateral preoptic region, and anterior thalamic nuclei to the medial habenulum. There is also input from the lateral hypothalamus, substantia innominata, midbrain raphe nuclei, ventral tegmentum, and superior cervical ganglia.

3. Output—to the **fasciculus retroflexus** to the interpeduncular nuclei and the midbrain raphe nuclei.

C. Pineal gland

1. **Pineal gland** (epiphysis)—attached to the roof of the third ventricle by ventral (posterior commissure) and dorsal (habenular commisure) commisures. It is composed of glia and pinealocytes that contain serotonin (5-HT) and CCK. It is related to neurosensory photoreceptors and secretes 5-HT (made in the pinealocytes), norepinephrine (made in the sympathetic neurons terminating there), melatonin, TRH, LHRH, and somatostatin (inhibits GH).

2. Melatonin—made from 5-HT and the daily levels fluctuate with diurnal light. Secretion decreases with more light in the day. An oversecreting pineal gland delays puberty. A hypofunctional pineal gland causes precocious puberty.

3. Bilateral lesions of the suprachiasmatic nuclei of the hypothalamus (which conveys retinal input to the pineal gland) abolish circadian rhythms of eating and drinking and the estrous cycle.

D. Thalamus (**Figs. A–25 and A–26**)

1. The internal medullary lamina separates the medial and lateral nuclear groups. The external medullary lamina is at the lateral border. The specific relay nuclei are in a defined specific pathway, whereas the association nuclei are not.

2. **Anterior nuclear group**—the anteroventral, anterodorsal, and anteromedial nuclei. Input is from the mamillothalamic tract and the fornix. Output is to the cingulate gyrus by way of the anterior limb of the IC. It has a role in regulating visceral function.

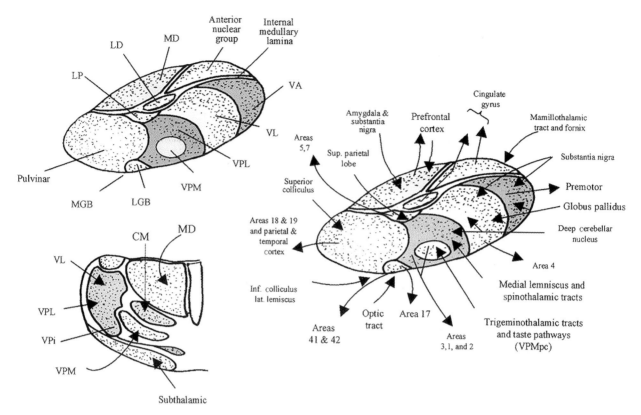

Figure A–25   Thalamic nuclei.

3. **Medio dorsal (MD) nuclear group**—between the internal medullary lamina and the periventricular gray. It functions to integrate somatic and visceral activities and to control affective behavior. It is disconnected with prefrontal lobotomies. Input is from the amygdala, orbitofrontal, and temporal cortex. Output is to the frontal association cortex or prefrontal area. Reciprocal connections exist with the frontal eye fields.

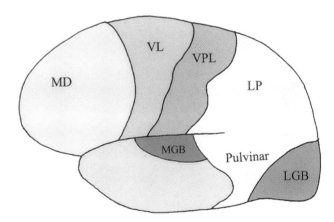

Figure A–26   Thalamocortical projections.

4. **Midline nuclei**—the periventricular gray and the massa intermedia. Output is to the amygdala and cingulate gyrus.

5. **Intralaminar nuclear group**—in the internal medullary lamina and has diffuse cortical projections. The **centro medial (CM) nucleus** had input from area 4 and output to the **putamen**. The **parafascicular nucleus** has input from area 6 and output to the **caudate**. The **rostral intralaminar nuclei** have input from the reticular formation and output to diffuse cortical areas. It acts as the **thalamic pacemaker** controlling cortical electrical activities and wakefulness.

6. Lateral nuclear group—the **lateral dorsal (LD) nucleus** which has output to the cingulum and supralimbic parietal lobe; the **lateral posterior (LP) nucleus** which has input from the parietal lobe and output to areas 5 and 7; and the **pulvinar**, which has input from the superior

colliculus, reciprocal connections with the **occipital cortex**, and also connects with the **temporal and parietal lobes**. Extrageniculate visual pathways go to the secondary visual areas. There are three visuotopic thalamocortical pathways because the LGB, inferior pulvinar, and the lateral pulvinar all go to areas 17, 18, and 19, respectively. The medial pulvinar may connect with the superior temporal gyrus.

7. Ventral nuclear group—the ventral anterior (VA), ventral lateral (VL), and ventral posterior (VP) nuclei, which are all relay nuclei. The caudal aspect carries specific sensory information and the rostral aspect has input from the striatum, cerebellum, and SN.

   (a) **VA** nucleus—involved with recruiting the cortical response like the intralaminar nuclei. The mamillothalamic tract passes through it. Input is from the **GP**, substantia nigra (SN), and areas 6 and 8. Output is to the **frontal cortex** and intralaminar nuclei.

   (b) **VL** nucleus pars oralis (VLo)—input from the **GP** and output to the **premotor and supplementary motor cortex**. The pars caudalis (VLc) has input from the **contralateral deep cerebellar nuclei and the red nuclei** and reciprocal connections with **area 4**.

   (c) VP nucleus—has (1) the VPLo with input from the contralateral deep cerebellar nuclei and output to the motor cortex; (2) the VPLc with input from the medial lemniscus (ML) and output to the sensory cortex (**limbs are lateral here and the back is dorsal**); (3) the VPM with input from the contralateral spinal and principal sensory nuclei of CN V and the ipsilateral dorsal trigeminal tract and output to the sensory cortex. The face has bilateral VPM representation. The taste fibers from the nucleus solitarius go to the central tegmental tract uncrossed to the VPMpc to the parietal operculum area 43; and (4) the VPI with output to the ipsilateral SII. The SII also gets bilateral input from the SI areas.

8. Posterior thalamic nuclear complex—input from the spinothalamic tract, ML, and SI. Output is to the retroinsular cortex and the posterior auditory cortex.

9. **Medial geniculate body (MGB)**—the auditory relay nucleus. It has input by means of the **inferior brachium** from the inferior colliculus and reciprocal connections with the primary auditory cortex with **spatial representation of tonal frequency**. It is tonotopic with high-frequency sounds medially. Heschl's gyrus is in the superior temporal convolution (area 41), where higher frequencies are still medial.

10. **Lateral geniculate body (LGB)**—the visual relay nucleus. It has six layers, with one and two being magnocellular and three to six parvicellular. It receives fibers of the contralateral visual field from the optic tract. **Crossed fibers from the contralateral eye go to layers 1, 4, and 6. Uncrossed fibers go to layers 2, 3, and 5.** Input is from the retinal ganglion cells. Reciprocal connections exist with the calcarine cortex 17 and pulvinar. **No binocular fusion** is present here because fibers from different eyes end in different layers. The **superior retina (inferior visual field) goes to the medial LGB** (90 degrees medial rotation).

11. **Thalamic reticular nuclei**—form a shell over the dorsal thalamus. They are a migrated derivative of the ventral thalamus and lie between the IC and the external medullary lamina. It samples passing fibers and gates the activity of the thalamus but has **no cortical projections**.

E. Miscellaneous

1. Neurotransmitters—most of the thalamus uses GABA as the output neurotransmitter. Input is usually excitatory with aspartate and glutamate from the deep cerebellar nuclei and the cortex.

2. Claustrum—has reciprocal connections with area 6 and input from the lateral hypothalamus, thalamic CM nucleus, and the locus ceruleus.

3. Thalamic radiations—the parts of the IC with reciprocal connections between the thalamus and cortex. The four thalamic peduncles are the **anterior**, with fibers from the medial and anterior thalamic nuclei to the frontal lobe; **superior**, with connections to the precentral and postcentral gyri; **posterior**, with connections to the calcarine cortex; and the **inferior** with connections to Heschl's gyrus.

F. Internal capsule (IC)

1. The IC has thalamic radiations and corticospinal, bulbar, reticular, and pontine fibers.

2. **Anterior limb**—contains the anterior thalamic peduncle and the prefrontal corticopontine tract.

3. **Genu**—contains the corticobulbar and corticoreticular tracts.

4. **Posterior limb**—contains the corticospinal tract, the superior thalamic peduncle, and the corticotectal/rubral/and reticular tracts. Motor fibers are anterior to sensory fibers here.

5. **Retrolenticular portion**—contains the posterior thalamic peduncle for visual information.

6. **Sublenticular IC**—contains the inferior thalamic peduncle for auditory information.

7. **Blood supply to the IC—by way of the lenticulostriate branches of the MCA (lateral and rostral aspects of the anterior and posterior limbs and genu), the recurrent artery of Heubner of the ACA (caudal anterior limb), the ICA perforators (genu), the anterior choroidal artery (caudal posterior limb and retrolenticular), and the PCOM (caudal posterior limb) (Figs. A–27 and A–28).**

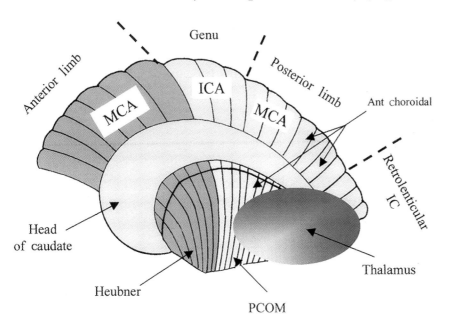

Figure A–27   Blood supply to the internal capsule.

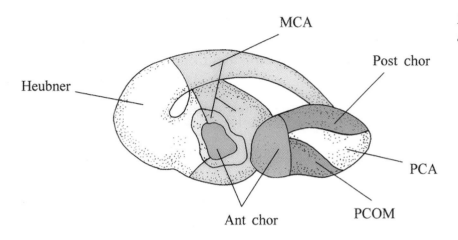

MCA

Post chor

Heubner

PCA

Ant chor

PCOM

Figure A–28   Blood supply to the thalamus and striatum.

X. BASAL GANGLIA

A. General information—the basal ganglia include the corpus striatum, the amygdala, the subthalamic nuclei, and the substantia nigra (SN). The neostriatum or **striatum is a telencephalic** structure and includes the caudate and putamen. The paleostriatum is a diencephalic structure and includes the globus pallidus (GP). The subthalamic nucleus is also a diencephalic structure. The archistriatum includes the amygdala and is from the telencephalon. The corpus striatum includes the neostriatum and the paleostriatum, which includes the caudate, putamen, and GP. The lentiform nuclei are the putamen and GP.

B. Caudate—composed of a head, body (separated from the thalamus by the stria terminalis and the terminal vein), and tail (in the roof of the temporal horn near the amygdala).

C. Nucleus accumbens septi—where the caudate and putamen meet anteriorly.

D. Afferent fibers to the basal ganglia system are to the striatum (caudate and putamen).

E. Striatal input—from the cortex, thalamic CM and parafascicular nuclei, SN, midbrain dorsal raphe nucleus, and the lateral amygdala. Corticostriate fibers are from area 4 to bilateral putamen, premotor cortex to the ipsilateral caudate and putamen, and the prefrontal cortex to the caudate. The amygdalostriate fibers go from the amygdala to the caudate and putamen and to the SI to the caudate. **The thalamostriate fibers are from the intralaminar CM nucleus to the putamen and the parafascicular nucleus (PF) to the caudate.** The nigrostriatal fibers are from the substantia nigra (SN) to the caudate and putamen with inhibitory dopamine (DA). The raphe nucleus sends inhibitory fibers to the striatum.

F. Striatal output—**inhibitory with GABA** to the medial GP to the ipsilateral thalamus and to the lateral GP with reciprocal connections to the subthalamic nucleus. Output is also to the **SN pars reticulata** to the superior colliculus, tegmentum, and the thalamic VA, VL, and MD with GABA.

G. The lateral medullary lamina is between the putamen and the GP. The medial medullary lamina divides the medial and lateral GP. The accessory medullary lamina divides the mGP into inner and outer segments.

H. Globus pallidus (GP) input—from the striatum with GABA and enkephalin to the (lateral) lGP and substance P to the (medial) mGP. Huntington's disease has decreased substance P and enkephalin in the GP and SN. Also, the **subthalamus lateral part has reciprocal fibers** sending glutamate to the lGP, and the medial part connects to the mGP.

I. GP output—four bundles: the ansa lenticularis, lenticular fasciculus, pallidotegmental fibers (these three are only from the mGP), and the pallidosubthalamic fibers.

> 1. **Ansa lenticularis**—from the mGP and passes around the IC to FFH1 (Forel's Field H1, the prerubral field).
>
> 2. **Lenticular fasciculus** (FFH2 fibers)—from the mGP and passes through the IC to join the ansa lenticularis in Forel's field and enters the thalamic fasciculus.
>
> 3. **Thalamic fasciculus** (FFH1 fibers)—made up of the joined ansa lenticularis, lenticular fasciculus, and the cerebellothalamic tract (fibers from the contralateral deep cerebellar nuclei) to the thalamic VA and VL. The pallidotegmental fibers are from the mGP to the Forel H fibers to the **pedunculopontine nucleus**.
>
> 4. **Pallidosubthalamic** fibers—from the lGP to the subthalamus (ST). There are also fibers from the mGP to the stria medullaris to the lateral habenulum. There are fibers from the GP to VA, VL, and CM.

J. Subthalamus (ST)—lateral to the hypothalamus and medial to the IC. The nuclei include the subthalamic nuclei, **the zona incerta**, and the nucleus of the tegmental fields of Forel. Fibers passing through include the ansa lenticularis, FFH2, FFH1, and the subthalamic fasciculus. The subthalamic nuclei are over the rostral SN and use **glutamate** as a neurotransmitter. Input is from the lGP, prefrontal, premotor, and motor cortex, the CM and PF thalamic nuclei, and the pedunculopontine nucleus. The output is to the GPm and GPl (mainly) and the SN. The subthalamic fasciculus is from the lGP to the ST to the mGP and lGP and passes through the peduncular IC. The zona incerta is the gray matter between the thalamic and lenticular fasciculi. Laterally it is continuous with the thalamic reticular nucleus. Input is from the motor cortex.

K. Substantia nigra (SN)—input from **the striatum** (to the SNpr, pigmented neurons), GP, ST, pedunculopontine nucleus, and the dorsal raphe nucleus. Output from the SNpc is to the striatum. Output from the SNpr is to the thalamus and pedunculopontine nucleus. **The SN does not have output to the GP.**

L. Corpus striatum—output inhibitory to the mGP and the SNpr that inhibit the thalamic output to premotor and supplementary motor cortex, but not to area 4.

M. Putamen circuit—involved with **discrete motor movements**. Fibers are from the motor and somatosensory cortices to putamen to GP to thalamus to supplementary motor cortex.

N. Caudate circuit—involved with **cognitive function**. Fibers are from the cortical association areas to caudate to GP to thalamus to prefrontal area.

O. The striatum has a reciprocal connection with the SN (to the SNpr and from the SNpc).

P. The GP has a reciprocal connection with the ST. **There are no afferent fibers from the cortex or the thalamus to the GP.** The GPl connects to the ST. The GPm sends fibers to the thalamus (VL, VA, and CM).

Q. The cortex to striatum fibers use glutamate. The putamen to GP fibers use GABA.

R. The SNpc inhibits the putamen that inhibits the GP that inhibits the thalamus.

XI. HYPOTHALAMUS

A. Hypothalmus—controls visceral, autonomic, endocrine, and emotional function. It extends from the anterior perforated substance and the optic chiasm to the optic tracts and the mamillary bodies. It has an anterior and posterior part, median and lateral eminences, and an infundibulum.

1. **Median eminence**—where the CNS interacts with the pituitary gland.

2. Preoptic area—the periventricular gray of the most rostral part of the third ventricle and contains the medial and lateral preoptic nuclei.

3. Lateral hypothalamic area—contains the lateral hypothalamic nucleus.

4. Medial hypothalamic area—contains the supraoptic region, the tuberal region, and the mamillary region, which is continuous with the periaqueductal gray.

5. Supraoptic region—contains the **paraventricular and supraoptic nuclei** which secrete **oxytocin and vasopressin**, the anterior hypothalamic nucleus, and the **suprachiasmatic nucleus** which acts as a biologic clock with bilateral afferent input from the retinas.

6. Tuberal region—where the fornix separates the hypothalamus into medial and lateral regions.

7. Mamillary region—the mamillary bodies and the posterior hypothalamic nuclei.

8. Rostral and lateral is the basal olfactory region, whereas medial is the septal region with the medial and lateral septal nuclei and the nucleus accumbens septi.

9. Input to the hypothalmus is from:

   (a) **Medial forebrain bundle**—from the basal olfactory areas, septal nuclei, periamygdala, and subiculum to the lateral preoptic and lateral hypothalmic areas.

   (b) **Fornix**—from the hippocampus, which divides at the anterior commissure into precommissural fibers to the septal nucleus, lateral preoptic nucleus, and the dorsal hypothalamus, and into postcommissural fibers to the medial mamillary nucleus and the anterior thalamic nucleus.

   (c) **Stria terminalis**—from the amygdala to the hypothalamus.

   (d) **Mamillary peduncle**—from the brain stem reticular formation to the lateral mamillary nucleus.

   (e) **Dorsal longitudinal fasciculus**—from the midbrain's central gray to the periventricular hypothalamus.

   (f) **Retinohypothalamic tract**—from retinal ganglion cells to both suprachiasmatic nuclei and various hypothalamic nuclei for circadian rhythms.

(g) Input is also from the nucleus solitarius rostral segment (taste) and caudal segment (visceral) to the medial (taste) and lateral (visceral) hypothalamus and from the midbrain raphe nucleus, pons parabrachial nucleus, locus ceruleus, LGB, and the thalamus.

(h) The main input is from the two oldest cortical areas: the pyriform cortex to the amygdala to the stria terminalis to the hypothalamus and the hippocampus to the fornix to the septum, and so forth. A loop is formed as the cingulate gyrus connects to the entorhinal cortex to the hippocampus to the hypothalamus to the anterior thalamic nucleus back to the cingulate gyrus.

10. Output from the hypothalmus is to:

   (a) **Medial forebrain bundle**—from the lateral hypothalmus to the hippocampus.

   (b) **Stria terminalis**—from the hypothalamus to the amygdala.

   (c) **Dorsal longitudinal fasciculus**—from the mamillary bodies to the midbrain tegmentum and central gray.

   (d) **Mamillothalamic tract**—to the anterior thalamic nucleus.

   (e) **Mamillotegmental tract**—to the midbrain ventral and dorsal tegmentum.

   (f) **Descending autonomic projections**—to the brain stem and spinal cord from the paraventricular, lateral hypothalamus, and posterior hypothalmus to dorsal X, nucleus solitarius, nucleus ambiguous, medulla, and spinal intermediolateral cell column.

   (g) **Supraoptichypophyseal tract**—from the supraoptic and paraventricular nuclei to the posterior pituitary gland to release oxytocin, vasopressin, CCK, enkephalins, glucagon, dynorphin, and angiotensin.

   (h) **Tuberohypophyseal tract—from the arcuate nucleus of the tuber region to the median eminence and infundibular stem**, where releasing hormones are secreted into fenestrated capillaries that feed the anterior pituitary gland. The hypophyseal portal system is formed by the superior (from the supraclinoid ICA) and the inferior hypophyseal arteries (from the cavernous ICA's meningohypophyseal trunk) which join in and around the pituitary stalk and form sinusoids that feed both the infundibulum and anterior pituitary gland.

11. **Parasympathetic control**—anterior and medial (ventromedial) hypothalamic nuclei.

12. **Sympathetic control**—posterior and lateral hypothalamic nuclei.

13. **Decreases body temperature**—anterior hypothalamic nucleus.

14. **Increases body temperature**—posterior hypothalamic nucleus.

15. **Satiety center**—medial hypothalamic nucleus.

16. **Feeding center**—lateral hypothalamic nucleus.

17. **Arousal center**—posterior hypothalamic nucleus.

B. Pituitary gland

    1. The sella is located in the sphenoid bone.

    2. Adenohypophysis (anterior pituitary lobe)—comprises 75% of the gland and is composed of:

        (a) Pars tuberalis (includes part of the infundibular stalk and median eminence of the hypothalamus)

        (b) Pars intermedia (small in humans)

        (c) Pars distalis (most of the gland). It receives no direct arterial supply.

    3. Neurohypophysis—the pars nervosa (posterior lobe), **infundibulum**, and the supraoptic and paraventricular nuclei. It is of **diencephalic origin**, whereas the adenohypophysis is from the ectoderm in the roof of the stomodeum. The blood supply is from the superior hypophyseal artery to the infundibular stalk and the inferior hypophyseal artery to the pars nervosa.

XII. OLFACTORY SYSTEM (ALSO SEE SECTION XV)

A. Olfactory sense—the only sense without a thalamic relay. It functions to help find food and mates and to avoid predators.

B. Rhinencephalon—the olfactory bulbs, tracts, tubercles, striae, and the anterior olfactory nucleus and pyriform cortex. It is **paleopallium** compared with the archipallium of the hippocampus, dentate gyrus, fasciolar gyrus, and the supracallosal gyrus.

C. **Olfactory receptors**—in the upper posterior nasal cavity and consist of epithelium with primary bipolar cells with kinocilium.

D. Olfactory nerve—a group of unmyelinated fibers extending through the cribriform plate to synapse with the **mitral cells** (second neurons) in the olfactory bulb. The mitral cells and tufted cells are gathered together to form glomeruli. **Granule cells there have no axons.** The neurotransmitters are **glutamate and aspartate**.

E. Olfactory bulb—connects to the olfactory tract to the lateral olfactory stria and gyrus or the medial olfactory stria and gyrus. The axons of the mitral and tufted cells form the lateral olfactory tract.

F. **Lateral olfactory stria** goes to:

    1. Anterior olfactory nucleus. Some fibers cross in the **anterior commissure** to the contralateral anterior nucleus and olfactory bulb to the internal granule cells.

    2. Olfactory tubercle

    3. Amygdala

    4. **Pyriform cortex to the entorhinal cortex** to the hippocampus, insula, and frontal lobe by way of the uncinate fasciculus.

5. Pyriform cortex to the amygdala, the lateral preoptic hypothalamus, and the nucleus of the diagonal band.

6. Pyriform cortex to the MD thalamic nucleus to the orbitofrontal cortex.

G. **Medial olfactory stria**—goes to the subcallosal area and the paraterminal gyrus of the septal area.

H. Primary olfactory cortex—the **pyriform cortex** (the lateral olfactory gyrus from the lateral olfactory stria to the amygdala) and the periamygdaloid cortex. The secondary olfactory cortex is the **entorhinal area** of the anterior parahippocampus (area 28), which is posterior to the primary cortex.

I. **Anterior perforated substance**—bounded by the medial and lateral olfactory stria anteriorly, by the optic tract medially, and posteriorly by the diagonal band of Broca. It transmits perforating vessels.

J. Septal area—the subcallosal area and the paraterminal gyrus.

K. The medial and lateral septal nuclei are rostral to the anterior commissure and the preoptic area. The medial septal nucleus becomes continuous with the nucleus and tract of the **diagonal band of Broca**, which extends to the amygdala. **Septal input** is from the fornix and the mamillary peduncle. **Output** is through the stria medullaris to the medial habenular nucleus, the medial forebrain bundle to the lateral hypothalamus and midbrain tegmentum, and the fornix to the hippocampus.

L. **Anterior commissure**—the anterior part connects the two olfactory bulbs and the posterior part, which is larger, connects the two GP, putamen, external capsules, claustrums, and inferior and middle frontal gyri.

XIII. HIPPOCAMPAL FORMATION (FIGS. A–29 AND A–30)

A. Hippocampal formation—the presubiculum, subiculum, prosubiculum, hippocampus, and dentate gyrus. All are archipallium with **three layers**. The inferior **parahippocampus is isocortex with six layers**.

B. **Indusium griseum**—the supracallosal gyrus and the medial and lateral longitudinal striae. They are the remnants of the hippocampus that course over the dorsal surface of the corpus callosum.

C. Input to the hippocampus

1. **Entorhinal cortex** to the hippocampus and dentate gyrus.

2. **Medial septal nucleus** to the fimbria.

3. **Cingulate gyrus** to the cingulum to the presubiculum/entorhinal cortex to the hippocampus.

D. Output—via the **fornix**. The hippocampus and the subicular cortex (presubiculum, subiculum, and postsubiculum) to the alveus to the fimbria to the two forniceal crura to the forniceal commissure to

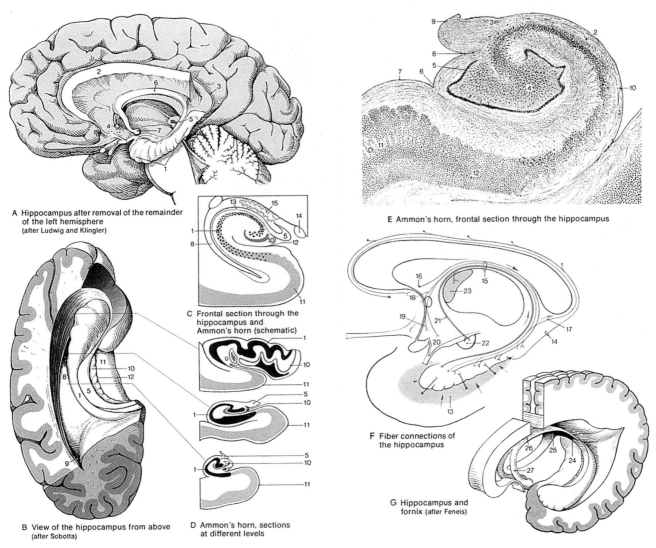

A Hippocampus after removal of the remainder
of the left hemisphere
(after Ludwig and Klingler)

B View of the hippocampus from above
(after Sobotta)

C Frontal section through the
hippocampus and
Ammon's horn (schematic)

D Ammon's horn, sections
at different levels

E Ammon's horn, frontal section through the hippocampus

F Fiber connections of
the hippocampus

G Hippocampus and
fornix (after Feneis)

Figure A–29   Hippocampus.

the body of the fornix under the corpus callosum to the separation at the rostral thalamus into anterior columns.

1. **Precommissural** fibers—go anterior to the interventricular foramen and rostral to the anterior commissure.

2. **Postcommissural** fibers—go anterior to the interventricular foramen and caudal to the anterior commissure. The subiculum projects to the postcommissural fornix (larger) to the medial nucleus of the mamillary body, the anterior thalamic nucleus, the lateral septal area of the rostral hypothalamus, the medial frontal cortex, and the cingulate and parahippocampal gyri. The hippocampus projects to the precommissural fornix to the caudal septal nucleus.

3. **Dentate fibers do not leave the hippocampus.** The **subiculum** may serve as the main output for the hippocampus and dentate gyrus. It is the sole direct cortical projector.

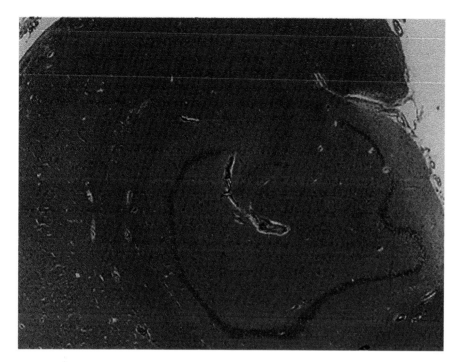

Figure A–30   Normal hippocampus (hematoxylin and eosin).

E. Function—the hippocampus has no olfactory function. Stimulation or lesioning causes psychomotor seizures. It is involved with recent memory, not remote. It helps to consolidate short-term memory into long-term memory. **Injury to the mamillary body and the fornix does not seem to impair memory.**

F. Papez circuit—suggested to be involved with emotion, combining the subjective, autonomic, and somatic elements. It is bidirectional and goes from the subiculum to the mamillary bodies to the mamillothalamic tract to the anterior thalamic nucleus to the entorhinal cortex to the subiculum.

G. Amygdala—merges caudally with the uncus of the parahippocampal gyrus.

    1. Input—from the lateral olfactory tract, pyriform cortex, hypothalamus, paraventricular thalamus, and the nucleus of the solitary tract to the lateral parabrachial nucleus to the amygdala. There is also input of noradrenergic fibers from the locus ceruleus, dopaminergic fibers from the SN and ventral tegmentum, cholinergic fibers from the substantia innominata and the lateral olfactory area, and serotonergic fibers from the raphe nucleus.

    2. Output

        (a) **Stria terminalis**—to mainly the nucleus of the stria terminalis at the caudate/thalamic junction to the hypothalamus.

        (b) Ventral amygdalofugal tract—from the amygdala and pyriform area to the lateral preoptic area, the septal area, the nucleus of the diagonal band, the substantia innominata (SI), the hippocampus, and the brain stem nuclei to regulate autonomic functions (with fear or stress).

        (c) Amygdalocortical

        (d) Amygdalostriate to the nucleus accumbens.

H. Amygdala stimulation—causes the arrest reaction and arousal with the initial reaction of flight, fear, and rage with pupillary dilation and growling. A stria terminalis injury does not change the response, but stimulation increases respiratory rate. If the ventral amygdalofugal fibers are damaged, no response occurs with stimulation.

I. Function—the amygdala serves as an interface between the cortex and the autonomic functions controlled by the hypothalamus and the brain stem. It dictates the emotion and the behavior for a specific situation. Much reciprocal cortical input and output are present.

J. **Substantia innominata or nucleus basalis of Meynert**—in the basal forebrain and extends from the olfactory tubercle to the hypothalamus. The subcommissural region contains the diagonal band of Broca, the anterior commissure, the median forebrain bundle (MFB), the ansa lenticularis, the ansa peduncularis, and the inferior thalamic peduncle. The substantia innominata input is from the amygdala, temporal lobe, pyriform cortex, and entorhinal cortex. Output is diffuse to the cortex. The substantia innominata has a high concentration of cholinergic neurons and is the **single major source of cholinergic fibers (ACh) to the cortex**. Cells degenerate here in Alzheimer's disease. Other cholinergic areas of the CNS are the **pedunculopontine nucleus**, the lateral dorsal tegmental nucleus, and the medial habenular nucleus.

K. Limbic system—controls behavior and emotion. It contains the amygdala, septal region, hypothalmus, epithalamus, thalamus, and medial tegmental region (**Fig. A–31**).

L. **C**-shaped structures—the limbic association areas, the hippocampus and fornix, the amygdala and stria terminalis, the caudate nucleus, and the lateral ventricles.

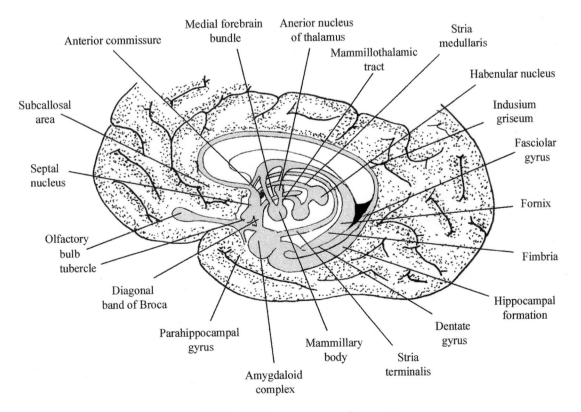

Figure A–31 Limbic structures and connections.

XIV. CEREBELLUM (FIGS. A–32—A–34)

A. Cerebellum—controls muscle tone, coordination, and equilibrium. It is divided into cortex/ medullary substance/intrinsic nuclei and hemisphere/vermis. Grossly it has many convolutions called folia. The three lobes are the anterior, posterior, and flocculonodular. In the vermis, there are 9 lobules: lingula, centralis, culmen, declive, folium, tuber, pyrimis, uvula, and nodulus.

1. Archicerebellum—the oldest section and contains the flocculus and nodulus. It is involved with vestibular function.

2. Paleocerebellum—the anterior lobe, which is rostral to the primary fissure (lingula, centralis, and culmen) and controls muscle tone with input from stretch receptors by means of the spinocerebellar tract.

3. Neocerebellum— the newest section, the posterior lobe between the primary fissure and the lateral fissures (declive, folium, tuber, pyrimis, and uvula). It controls coordination with input from the contralateral cortex by way of the pontine relay nuclei.

B. Cerebellar cortical layers—molecular (most superficial), Purkinje, and granular.

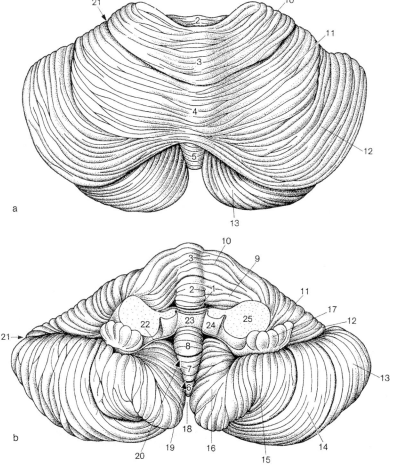

Figure A–32   Cerebellum surface anatomy.
a) Superior view. b) View from in front (cerebellar peduncles severed)

1–8	*Vermis*
1	Lingula
2	Central lobule
3	Culmen
4	Declive
5	Tuber
6	Pyramid
7	Uvula
8	Nodulus
9–17	*Cerebellar hemisphere*
9	Ala of central lobule
10	Quadrangular lobule
11	Lobulus simplex
12	Superior semilunar lobule
13	Inferior semilunar lobule
14	Paramedian lobule
15	Biventral lobule
16	Tonsil
17	Flocculus
18	Vallecula
19	Secondary fissure
20	Dorsolateral fissure
21	Primary fissure
22	Inferior medullary velum
23	Superior medullary velum
24	Superior cerebellar peduncle
25	Middle and inferior cerebellar peduncles

1. The molecular layer—contains basket cells (inibitory, −) and outer stellate cells (−). Axons from each basket cell touch 10 Purkinje's cells.

2. Purkinje cell layer—contains Purkinje's cells (−) that use GABA as the neurotransmitter. These were the first neurons identified in 1837. The myelinated axons synapse with the deep nuclei and the lateral vestibular nucleus and send collateral fibers to synapse on the Golgi's type II cells and excite the system. Purkinje's cells have the only myelinated axons in the cerebellum.

3. Granular layer—contains granule cells (excitatory, +, **glutamate**) and Golgi's type II cells (−). The granule cells supply four to five dendrites to form a glomerulus. It sends unmyelinated axons up to the molecular layer that bifurcate into **parallel fibers** that contact Purkinje's cell dendrites. The Golgi's type II cells have axons that synapse in the glomeruli of the granular layer and dendrites that extend to the molecular layer, where they synapse with parallel fibers.

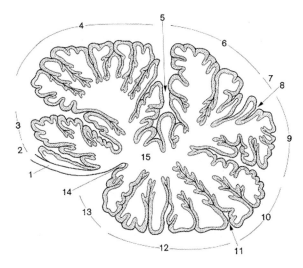

Figure A–33   Cerebellum median section.

1 Superior medullary velum
2 Lingula of cerebellum
3 Central lobule
4 Culmen
5 Primary fissure
6 Declive
7 Folium of vermis
8 Horizontal fissure
9 Tuber of vermis
10 Pyramid of vermis
11 Secondary fissure
12 Uvula of vermis, separated from nodulus by dorsolateral fissure
13 Nodulus
14 Fastigium
15 Corpus medullare

Figure A–34   Cerebellar functional zones.

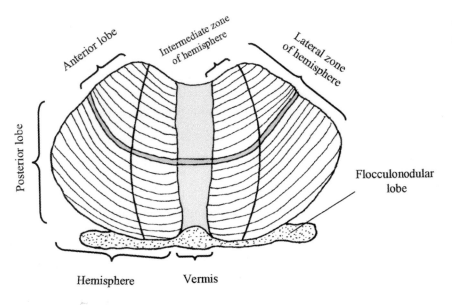

4. Afferent fibers to the cerebellar cortex—arrive by way of the superior, middle, and inferior cerebellar peduncles and are from the spinocerebellar, cuneocerebellar, olivocerebellar, vestibulocerebellar, and pontocerebellar tracts. These fibers lose their myelin in the cortex and end as mossy or climbing fibers.

C. Four spinocerebellar tracts exist:

1. Dorsal spinocerebellar tract—conveys proprioception from the joints, muscle spindles, and Golgi tendon organs from the lower extremities and upper trunk ipsilaterally to **Clarke's nucleus** in lamina VII in the intermediate zone of the spinal cord. From here the fibers enter the **inferior cerebellar peduncle** to the vermis and intermediate zone of the cerebellum and the fastigial and interposed nuclei.

2. Ventral spinocerebellar tract—conveys efference copies of motor commands reaching the alpha motor neurons and exteroceptive and proprioceptive information for the lower extremities. The initial cell bodies are "spinal border cells" in the anterior and intermediate horns. The tract ascends bilaterally, crosses in the spinal cord, enters the **superior cerebellar peduncle**, and crosses partly again in the cerebellum but is **mainly contralateral**.

3. Cuneocerebellar tract—the upper extremity equivalent to the dorsal spinocerebellar tract. It conveys **proprioception of the upper extremities** in the fasciculus cuneatus but synapses in the **accessory cuneate nucleus** in the caudal medulla above the cuneate nucleus and then enters the **inferior cerebellar peduncle ipsilaterally**.

4. Rostral spinocerebellar tract—the upper extremity equivalent to the ventral spinocerebellar tract. It provides internal feedback, ipsilateral, and enters the inferior cerebellar peduncle.

D. **Mossy fibers** (+)—from the spinocerebellar, pontocerebellar, and vestibulocerebellar tracts to the **granular layer** to **form the center of a glomerulus** with a mossy fiber rosette (up to 44 connections per fiber). The glomerulus contains one mossy fiber rosette (+), up to 20 dendrites of granule cells, and Golgi's type II cell's axons and dendrites. The mossy fiber stimulates the granule cells, whereas Golgi's type II cells inhibit them for feedback.

E. **Climbing fibers** (+, glutamate)—from the **contralateral inferior olivary complex** to the **molecular layer**, where they synapse on **Purkinje's cell dendrites**, granule cell parallel fibers (that stimulate Purkinje's cells), and other inhibitory cells such as basket and stellate cells (to silence the background). Climbing fibers may synapse with more than one cell. If the fiber discharges, so does the Purkinje's cell (all or none response).

F. All the cerebellar cells are inhibitory except granule cells, climbing fibers, and mossy fibers.

G. Deep nuclei—have neurons that release excitatory neurotransmitters aspartate and glutamate. There are four paired nuclei: fastigial (medial), globose, emboliform, and dentate (lateral).

1. Fastigial nucleus—in the midline roof of the fourth ventricle and sends fibers to the vestibular system bilaterally.

2. Globose and emboliform nuclei—called the nucleus interpositus and are involved with tone.

3. Dentate nucleus—the largest and shaped like a bag that is open medially toward the superior cerebellar peduncle. It is involved with coordination.

H. Corticonuclear projections—bidirectional and unilateral. They include the vermis-fastigial nucleus, paravermian zone-interposed nucleus, and hemisphere-dentate nucleus.

I. The deep nuclei project to the granular layer.

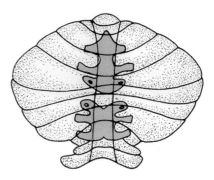

Figure A–35   Cerebellar homunculus.

J. Extracerebellar input to the deep nuclei can overcome the tonic inhibition by the cortex. Stimulation comes from the pons, inferior olivary nucleus, trigeminal sensory nucleus, reticulotegmental tract, locus ceruleus, and raphe nucleus by climbing and mossy fibers. The pons sends crossed and uncrossed fibers to the dentate nuclei. Within the inferior olivary complex, the principal olivary nucleus sends crossed fibers to the dentate nucleus, the medial and dorsal accessory olivary nuclei send crossed fibers to the interposed nucleus, and the medial accessory olive sends crossed fibers to the fastigial nucleus. The red nucleus sends crossed fibers to the interposed nucleus.

K. There is somatotopic organization with touch ipsilateral in the anterior lobe and bilateral in the posterior lobe. Audiovisual information is in the midline (**Fig. A–35**).

L. Afferent fibers to the cerebellum—enter mainly through the middle and inferior cerebellar peduncles. They outnumber efferent fibers 40 : 1.

1. Inferior cerebellar peduncle

(a) **Restiform body**—contains only afferent fibers from the **inferior olivary complex and pons**.

(b) **Juxtarestiform body**—medial to the restiform body, contains afferent and efferent fibers from the **vestibular system** to the uvula, nodulus, and fastigial nucleus.

2. Middle cerebellar peduncle—contains only afferent fibers. The cerebral cortex to the ipsilateral pons to the contralateral cerebellar hemisphere (**corticopontine fibers**) and to both sides of the vermis as mossy fibers. The nodulus is the only part of the cerebellum without pontine input.

3. Superior cerebellar peduncle—receives afferent fibers from the **ventral spinocerebellar tract**. It also has efferent fibers.

M. Efferent fibers—mainly from the deep nuclei and most leave through the superior cerebellar peduncle.

1. Inferior peduncle (through the **juxtarestiform body**)

(a) Fastigial nucleus to the contralateral reticular nucleus, pons, and spinal cord and bilateral lateral and inferior vestibular nuclei.

(b) Vermian cortex and flocculonodular lobe (through Purkinje's fibers that bypass the deep nuclei) to the ipsilateral vestibular nuclei. The flocculus sends fibers to the superior and medial vestibular nuclei. The nodulus and uvula send fibers to the superior, medial, and inferior vestibular nuclei. The vestibular nuclei also receive input from the fastigial nuclei. The vestibulocerebellar feedback is to the uvula and flocculonodular lobes.

2. Superior peduncle

(a) **Dentate nucleus** to the **contralateral thalamic VL**, **VPLo**, and centrolateral (CL) nuclei to the cortex. This controls coordination. An ipsilateral cerebellar lesion causes ipsilateral dyscoordination because it controls the contralateral cerebral cortex.

(b) **Interposed nucleus to the contralateral red nucleus** (some to the thalamus VL and VA) crossing back to the ipsilateral spinal cord for ipsilateral tone control.

(c) The dentate nucleus sends crossed fibers to the principal olive, the emboliform nucleus to the dorsal accessory olive, and the globose nucleus to the medial accessory olive.

N. Organization

1. Vermian zone—the Purkinje's fibers inhibit the vestibular nuclei to decrease extensor muscle tone. The fastigial nucleus gets ipsilateral inhibition from the vermis and gives bilateral stimulation to the vestibular nuclei, pons, medulla, thalamus, and cervical spine. It controls posture, tone, equilibrium, and locomotion.

2. Paramedian zone—sends fibers to the interposed nucleus to the thalamus and red nucleus for ipsilateral flexor tone.

3. Lateral zone—includes the hemispheres and sends fibers to the dentate nucleus to the thalamic VL and VPLo to the motor 4 for ipsilateral coordination. This is the largest efferent pathway.

O. Functional considerations

1. Cerebellar lesions—produce ipsilateral deficits that gradually attenuate with time. Injuries to the superior cerebellar peduncle and the dentate nucleus cause the most severe and persistent deficits.

2. SCA syndrome (lateral superior pontine syndrome)—causes ipsilateral ataxia, nystagmus, paresis of conjugate gaze, Horner's syndrome, contralateral decreased pain and temperature in the face and body, and proprioception in the lower $>$ upper extremities, dizziness, nausea, and vomiting.

3. AICA syndrome (lateral inferior pontine syndrome)—causes ipsilateral nystagmus, facial paralysis, conjugate gaze paralysis, deafness and tinnitus, ataxia, decreased facial sensation, contralateral decreased pain and temperature sensation in the body, nausea, vomiting, and vertigo.

4. PICA syndrome (lateral medullary syndrome, Wallenberg's syndrome)—causes ipsilateral loss of pain sensation and numbness in the face, ataxia, nystagmus, Horner's syndrome, dysphagia, hoarseness, decreased sensation in the extremities, contralateral decreased pain and temperature in the body, nausea, vomiting, and hiccups.

5. Neocerebellar lesions (posterior lobe)—affect skilled voluntary movement. Lesions cause hypotonia, fatiguability, pendular and sluggish deep tendon reflexes (DTRs), asynergia with decreased

coordination, dysmetria, dysdiadokinesis, rebound with the arm hitting the chest when dropped, decomposition of movement breaking a task into multiple acts, intention tremor (mainly proximal), ataxia of axial muscles, nystagmus when looking to a lesion, and slow dysarthric speech.

6. Paleocerebellar lesions (anterior lobe)—cause transcient increased extensor tone. The anterior lobe normally inhibits the lateral vestibular nucleus and the reticular formation to tonically decrease extensor tone. Stimulation of the interposed nucleus to the red nucleus elicits ipsilateral limb flexion.

7. Archicerebellar lesions of the posterior vermis and flocculus—cause truncal ataxia and equilibrium disorders.

XV. CRANIAL NERVES (FIG. A–36)

A. General information—cranial nerves carry fibers of six different modalities.

1. General somatic efferent (GSE) fibers—innervate muscles that develop from somites (CNs III, IV, VI, XII).

2. Special visceral efferent (SVE) fibers or branchial fibers—innervate muscles from the branchial arches (CNs V, VII, IX, X, XI).

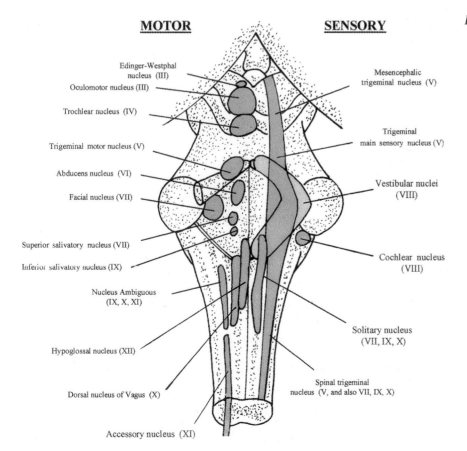

Figure A–36   Cranial nerve nuclei.

3. General visceral efferent (GVE) fibers—innervate the viscera, glands, and smooth muscle (CNs III, VII, IX, X).

4. General somatic efferent (GSA) fibers—transmit somatic sensation from the head, neck, sinuses, and meninges (CNs V, VII, IX, X).

5. Visceral efferent (VA) fibers—transmit visceral information but not pain impulses (CNs IX, X).

6. Special efferent (SA) fibers—transmit smell, vision, taste, balance, and hearing (CNs I, II, VII, IX, VIII).

B. Cranial nerve I (olfactory nerve)

1. SA—the neurosensory cells in the olfactory epithelium are the primary neurons and also serve as the sensory receptors (unlike other special sensory nerves that have separate receptors). These cells send 20 bundles of axons (the olfactory nerves proper) across the cribriform plate of the ethmoid bone to synapse on the secondary neurons in the olfactory bulb, the **mitral cells** (go to the lateral olfactory area), and the **tufted cells** (go to the anterior olfactory nucleus, lateral, intermediate, and medial olfactory areas). The olfactory tract carries these secondary neuron axons to:

   (a) The lateral olfactory stria to the lateral (primary) olfactory area, which consists of the uncus, entorhinal area (anterior part of the hippocampal gyrus), limen insula (junction of insular and frontal lobe cortex), and part of the amygdaloid cortex. The pear-shaped area containing the uncus, entorhinal area, and limen insula is the **pyriform cortex**.

   (b) The intermediate olfactory stria to the anterior perforated substance (intermediate olfactory area) between the olfactory trigone and optic tract.

   (c) The medial olfactory stria to the medial olfactory area (septal area) in the subcallosal region of the medial frontal lobe, which mediates the emotional response to odors with its limbic connections.

2. **Diagonal band of Broca—connects all three olfactory areas.**

3. **Anterior olfactory nucleus**—located between the olfactory bulb and tract and it receives fibers from the tufted cells and sends axons to either (1) the anterior commissure to the contralateral olfactory bulb or (2) the ipsilateral olfactory cortical areas.

4. Efferent fibers from the olfactory areas travel in:

   (a) The medial forebrain bundle from all three olfactory areas to the hypothalamus.

   (b) The stria medullaris thalami from the olfactory areas to the habenular nucleus.

   (c) The stria terminalis from the amygdala to the anterior hypothalamus and preoptic area. The hypothalamus sends the olfactory information to the reticular formation, salivatory nuclei, and dorsal motor nucleus of X (to cause nausea, acceleration of peristalsis, and increased gastric secretion).

C. Cranial nerve II (optic nerve)

1. SA—Bipolar cells of the retina (the primary sensory neurons) connect to the ganglion cells (secondary neurons). There are three types of retinal ganglion cells:

    (a) X cells—have the largest cell bodies, with slower transmission, and produce a tonic response to the LGB and pretectum.

    (b) Y cells—have rapid transmission, and produce a phasic response to the LGB and superior colliculus.

    (c) W cells—have the smallest cell bodies, very slow transmission, produce both tonic and phasic responses to the superior colliculus and pretectum.

2. Ganglion cells—send axons to the optic nerve (really a tract and not a nerve) through the optic canal to the optic chiasm to the optic tract to (1) the thalamic LGB for conscious vision, (2) the pretectal area for the light reflex, (3) the superior colliculus for eye movement reflexes, and (4) both suprachiasmatic nuclei for neuroendocrine function.

3. LGB—has tertiary neurons that form the optic radiations to the primary visual cortex surrounding the calcarine fissure. The visual image is inverted by the lens, and fibers from the right visual field cross to the left retina and end up in the left cortex. These fibers from the right eye cross to the left optic tract in the chiasm and fibers from the left eye stay on the left side traveling through the left optic nerve and tract.

4. **Meyer's loop**—courses anteriorly toward the temporal pole before turning posteriorly and carries fibers from the contralateral superior visual quadrant.

5. **Von Willebrand's knee**—contains fibers crossing from the contralateral optic nerve that travel a short distance into the other optic nerve before continuing through the optic tract.

D. Cranial nerve III (oculomotor nerve)

1. GSE—the oculomotor nuclear complex is at the level of the superior colliculus and has subnuclei that supply individual muscles. The lateral subnuclei supply the ipsilateral inferior rectus, inferior oblique, and medial rectus. The medial subnucleus supplies the contralateral superior rectus. The central subnucleus in the midline supplies the levator palpebrae superioris bilaterally.

    (a) The lower motor nerve (LMN) axons—course through the tegmentum of the midbrain through the red nucleus and medial aspect of the cerebral peduncles to enter the interpeduncular cistern at the midbrain/pons junction.

    (b) The nerve passes between the PCA and SCA, enters the oculomotor trigone in the posterior roof of the cavernous sinus, through the superior orbital fissure, through the anulus of Zinn, and into the orbit, where it divides into superior and inferior divisions. The superior division ascends lateral to the optic nerve to supply the superior rectus and levator palpebrae superioris muscles. The inferior division supplies the inferior rectus, inferior oblique, and medial rectus muscles.

    (c) Parasympathetic fibers—travel with the inferior division and may branch off directly or from the nerve to the inferior oblique muscle to enter the ciliary ganglion.

2. GVE—the **Edinger-Westphal nucleus** is in the midbrain superior to the oculomotor complex. Its fibers travel with CN III (on the dorsal superficial aspect) until it branches from the inferior oblique branch in the orbit and terminates in the ciliary ganglion near the apex of the cone of the extraocular muscles. Postganglionic fibers form 6 to 10 **short ciliary nerves** that travel with branches of V1 to enter the rear of the eye near the optic nerve and travel forward between the choroid and sclera to terminate in the ciliary body and iris. They control the pupillary constrictor muscle to cause pupillary constriction and the ciliary muscles to cause lens bending for accommodation.

E. Cranial nerve IV (the trochlear nerve)

1. GSE—the trochlear nucleus is at the level of the inferior colliculus. It gives rise to the trochlear nerve, which **crosses in the superior medullary velum** of the midbrain behind the aqueduct, exits the contralateral side just below the inferior colliculus, courses around the peduncles, emerges between the PCA and SCA with CN III, travels in the lateral wall of the cavernous sinus, through the superior orbital fissure, into the orbit above the anulus of Zinn, crosses medially near the roof of the orbit over the levator palpebrae and superior rectus muscles to innervate the contralateral superior oblique muscle. It causes inward and downward rotation of the eye (intortion). The trochlear nerve is the smallest cranial nerve, the only to exit from the dorsum of the brain stem, the only nerve in which all LMN axons decussate, the only nerve to deccusate outside of the CNS, and the CN with the longest intracranial course.

F. Cranial nerve V (the trigeminal nerve) (**Fig. A–37**)

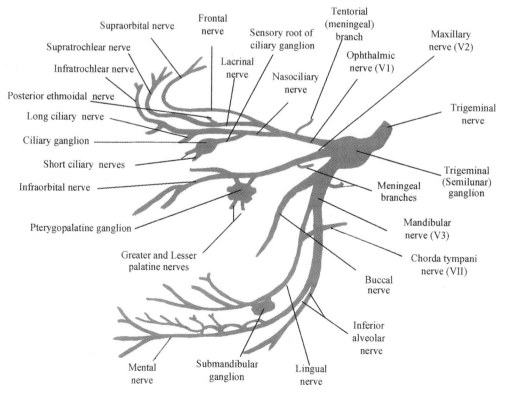

Figure A–37   Trigeminal nerve schema.

1. The trigeminal nerve leaves the midlateral surface of the pons as a large sensory root (**portio major**) and a smaller motor root (**portio minor**). The sensory ganglion (semilunar, gasserian, or trigeminal ganglion) lies in Meckel's cave on the floor of the middle fossa.

    (a) Three nerve divisions—the ophthalmic (V1), maxillary (V2), and mandibular (V3), which exit the skull through the superior orbital fissure, foramen rotundum, and foramen ovale, respectively.

    (b) Nerve branches—the V1 branches are the lacrimal, frontal, nasociliary (with long and short ciliary nerves), and the meningeal branch to the dura of the anterior and middle cranial fossa. The V2 branches are the zygomatic, infraorbital (with superior alveolar nerves), pterygopalatine, and meningeal nerves to the anterior and middle fossa. The V3 branches are the buccal, auriculotemporal, lingual, inferior alveolar, meningeal to anterior and middle fossa, and multiple motor branches.

    (c) Sympathetic fibers to the orbit—travel with the ICA and then with the **long and short ciliary nerves** from V1 to the eye.

    (d) Parasympathetic fibers from the ciliary ganglion—travel with the short ciliary nerves (that pass through the ciliary ganglion without synapsing) to the eye.

2. SVE—the Motor nucleus of V sends fibers to V3 (mandibular branch) to supply the muscles of mastication (masseter, temporalis, medial and lateral pterygoids), the **tensor tympani, the tensor veli palatini, the mylohyoid, and the anterior belly of the digastric muscle** (the posterior belly is supplied by CN VII). The branches to the tensor veli palatini and the tensor tympani pass through the otic ganglion without synapsing.

3. GSA—sensation to the face, forehead, nose, mouth, teeth, and dura of anterior and middle fossae. Fibers from V1 (ophthalmic branch), V2 (maxillary branch), and V3 (mandibular branch) to the trigeminal ganglion to the spinal trigeminal tract to the spinal trigeminal nucleus to the ventral (crossed) and dorsal (uncrossed, mainly V3) trigeminothalamic tracts to the thalamic VPM.

    (a) The **spinal trigeminal nucleus** is for pain and temperature and some touch. The **principal sensory nucleus** of CN V is for touch and pressure. The **mesencephalic nucleus** of CN V is for proprioception of the jaw and eyes.

    (b) **Ventral trigeminothalamic tract**—crossed and mainly involved with pain and touch and pressure.

    (c) **Dorsal trigeminothalamic tract**—uncrossed and mainly involved with touch and pressure.

4. Spinal trigeminal nucleus—consists of three parts (pars oralis, pars interpolaris, and pars caudalis). It extends from the pons to C2. Rostrally it merges with the primary sensory nucleus of CN V and caudally with the substantia gelatinosa of C2. There is also input from CN VII, IX, and X.

5. V1 fibers lie ventral and V3 fibers dorsal in the trigeminal nerve, although there is medial rotation of the nerve after the ganglion.

6. The pars oralis extends from the pons to the hypoglossal nucleus and covers the nose and mouth. The pars interpolaris extends down to the obex and covers the face. The pars caudalis extends down to C2, covers the forehead, jaw, and cheek, and is where most pain fibers synapse.

7. Mesencephalic nucleus—contains primary neurons, and the fibers travel with the motor root (portio minor).

8. Trigeminal reflexes—corneal from CN V1 to VII to cause bilateral blinking and to CN III to cause elevation of the eyes (Bell's phenomenon); tearing from V1 to the superior salivatory nucleus; salivation from CN V to the inferior salivatory nucleus; sneezing from CN V to the nucleus ambiguous to the respiratory center of the reticular formation, phrenic nerves, and intercostal muscles; vomiting from CN V to X; and jaw jerking (masseter) from mesencephalic nucleus to LMN of temporalis and masseter muscles.

G. Cranial nerve VI (the abducens nerve)

1. GSE—the abducens nucleus is just ventral to the fourth ventricle in the pontine tegmentum. Axons course ventrally and emerge at the pontomedullary junction just lateral to the pyramid. The nerve travels in the subarachnoid space of the posterior fossa, bends over the petrous apex, and goes through **Dorello's canal** to enter the cavernous sinus. It travels just lateral to the ICA in the cavernous sinus, enters the orbit at the medial end of the superior orbital fissure, goes through the anulus of Zinn (tendinous ring), and innervates the lateral rectus muscle.

    (a) The nucleus serves as the **horizontal gaze center** and has both motor fibers to the ipsilateral lateral rectus muscle and interneurons to the medial longitudinal fasciculus (MLF) to the contralateral medial rectus muscle.

    (b) There is afferent input from the medial vestibular nucleus, the parapontine reticular formation (PPRF), the reticular formation, and the nucleus prepositus.

    (c) A lesion of this nerve causes impaired ipsilateral lateral gaze, whereas a nuclear lesion impairs ipsilateral gaze of both eyes.

    (d) It is the most frequently injured CN because of its long intracranial course. The center for vertical gaze is the rostral interstitial nucleus of the medial longitudinal fasciculus (MLF) between the midbrain and diencepahlon. The horizontal and vertical gaze centers are connected by the PPRF.

H. Cranial nerve VII (the facial nerve) (**Fig. A–38**)

1. SVE—the facial motor nucleus in the pontine tegmentum sends axons dorsally toward the fourth ventricle that loop around the CN VI nucleus (forming the facial colliculus) and then travel ventrally to emerge from the pontomedullary junction between the CN VI and VIII.

    (a) The nervus intermedius is lateral to the motor facial branch at the brain stem. The facial nerve then goes with CN VIII through the internal acoustic meatus to the petrous temporal bone. The axons travel in the facial canal between the cochlea and vestibular organs and then turn laterally and caudally.

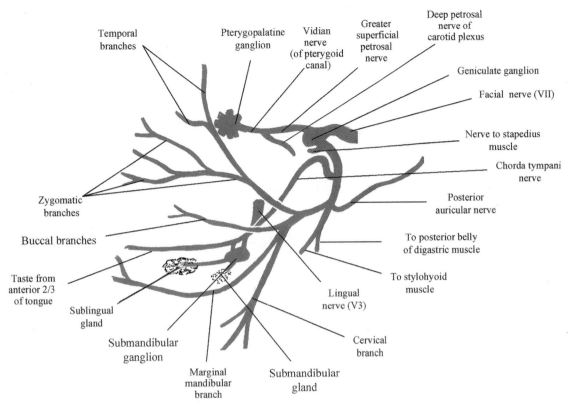

Figure A–38   Facial nerve schema.

(b) The first muscle branch is to the **stapedius muscle**. The branchial motor fibers then exit the facial canal at the stylomastoid foramen and immediately innervate the **stylohyoid, posterior belly of the digastric**, and the occipitalis muscles.

(c) The remaining fibers travel in the substance of the parotid gland to innervate the muscles of facial expression, platysma, and buccinator.

2. GVE, GSA, and SVA fibers travel in the **nervus intermedius**, which exits the brain stem between the motor branch of CN VII and VIII.

3. GVE—the **superior salivatory nucleus** sends axons to the nervus intermedius to (1) the **greater superficial petrosal nerve** to the **pterygopalatine ganglion** to the lacrimal gland for lacrimation and the mucosa of the nose and mouth for secretion; and (2) the **chorda tympani nerve** that joins with the lingual nerve (V3) to the **submandibular ganglion** to the submandibular and sublingual glands for salivation.

(a) The olfactory areas and the limbic system send input to the hypothalamus which influences the superior salivatory nucleus by way of the dorsal longitudinal fasciculus.

(b) Greater superficial petrosal nerve—exits the petrous temporal bone by way of the greater petrosal foramen to the middle fossa, passes deep to the trigeminal ganglion and down the foramen lacerum to the pterygoid canal (vidian canal), where it joins with the deep petrosal nerve (sympathetic fibers from the plexus that surrounds the ICA) to form the **nerve of the pterygoid canal**. This nerve goes to the pterygopalatine fossa where the pterygopalatine ganglion is suspended from the V2 nerve. Fibers from this ganglia travel with V2 to the lacrimal gland and the mucosa of the nose and mouth.

(c) Chorda tympani nerve—exits the petrotympanic fissure to join the lingual branch of V3 1 cm below the foramen ovale to the submandibular gland that is suspended from the lingual nerve.

4. GSA—sensation of the external auditory meatus and the back of the ear is carried to the geniculate ganglion (at the facial genu in the petrous bone) to the spinal trigeminal tract.

5. SVA—taste in the **anterior $\frac{2}{3}$ of the tongue** travels in the chorda tympani nerve to the geniculate ganglion to the rostral nucleus solitarius.

6. The first branch of the facial nerve is the greater superficial petrosal nerve (just before the geniculate ganglion), followed by the nerve to the stapedius, the chorda tympani, and the motor branches ("ten zebras bit my clock"—Temporal, Zygomatic, Buccal, Mandibular, and Cervical branches).

7. Bell's palsy (CN VII dysfunction)—causes ipsilateral face weakness, decreased sensation and taste, impaired salivation and lacrimation, and hyperacusis.

8. Upper half of face—receives bilateral innervation, so central facial palsy involves only the contralateral lower face.

9. There is memetic or emotional innervation such that involuntary contraction of the face can occur with emotion even after a corticobulbar fiber lesion.

I. Cranial nerve VIII (the vestibulocochlear nerve) (**Fig. A–39**)

1. SSA—hearing is detected in the **organ of Corti**, which sends fibers to the **spiral ganglion** (first neuron, at the modiolus in the center of the cochlea) to the cochlear nerve to the ventral (crossed and uncrossed) and dorsal (uncrossed) cochlear nuclei (second neuron) to the ventral (**trapezoid body**), intermediate, and dorsal acoustic striae (mostly crossed) to the **lateral lemniscus** to the **inferior colliculus** (third neuron) to the **MGB** (fourth neuron) to the temporal lobe (fifth neuron). The ventral cochlear nucleus also sends fibers to the reticular formation, the trapezoid body enroute to the superior olivary complex (the third neuron in this path), and the lateral lemniscus and its nucleus. The dorsal cochlear nucleus is involved with high frequencies and the ventral cochlear nucleus with low frequencies.

2. A lesion of the lateral lemniscus causes mainly contralateral deafness, although true unilateral deafness is generally due to a lesion of CN VIII or more distal.

3. Suppression of auditory input is by means of the olivocochlear bundle. The acoustic reflexes include the **superior olivary complex** to (1) both motor CN VII nuclei to the stapedius muscles to decrease the amplitude of the sound waves by reducing the movement of the ossicles,

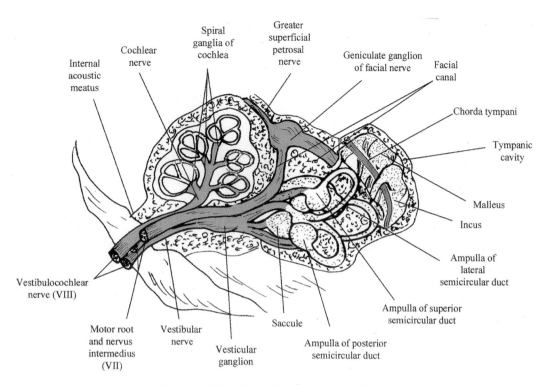

Internal acoustic meatus

Cochlear nerve

Spiral ganglia of cochlea

Greater superficial petrosal nerve

Geniculate ganglion of facial nerve

Facial canal

Chorda tympani

Tympanic cavity

Malleus

Incus

Ampulla of lateral semicircular duct

Ampulla of superior semicircular duct

Vestibulocochlear nerve (VIII)

Motor root and nervus intermedius (VII)

Vestibular nerve

Vesticular ganglion

Saccule

Ampulla of posterior semicircular duct

Figure A–39   Vestibulocochlear nerve schema.

and (2) both motor CN V nuclei to the tensor tympani muscles to decrease the sensitivity of the tympanic membrane by pulling it taught.

4. SSA—**Semicircular canals, utricle, and saccule** send fibers to the superior and inferior ganglia to CN VIII to the superior, inferior, medial, and lateral vestibular nuclei to:

   (a) Uncrossed fibers by way of the **juxtarestiform body** to the vestibulocerebellum.

   (b) The vestibulospinal tract to LMNs to facilitate extensors.

   (c) The MLF to the nuclei of CN III, IV, VI, PPRF, superior colliculus, and the interstitial nucleus of Cajal.

   (d) The hair cells for feedback modification.

5. The lateral vestibular nucleus (**Dieter's nucleus**)—sends axons to the ipsilateral lateral vestibulospinal tract to innervate antigravity extensors. The medial, superior, and inferior vestibular nuclei give rise to the medial vestibulospinal tract, which descends bilaterally to the cervical segments of the spinal cord. The medial and inferior vestibular nuclei have reciprocal connections with the cerebellum.

6. All nuclei contribute to the MLF. The descending part of the MLF continues as the medial vestibulospinal tract to the cervical LMNs. The utricle sends fibers to the superior vestibular ganglion to the lateral vestibular nucleus. The saccule sends fibers to the inferior vestibular ganglion to the inferior vestibular nucleus. The superior vestibular nucleus (sends uncrossed fibers) and the medial vestibular nucleus (sends crossed fibers) are mainly involved with co-ordination of eye movements with head movements.

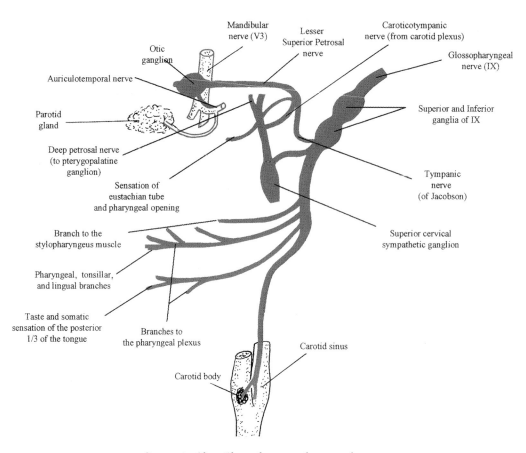

Figure A–40   Glossopharyngeal nerve schema.

7. Vestibular damage—causes decreased equilibrium, vertigo, and nystagmus.

8. Unilateral MLF damage rostral to the CN VI nucleus causes weakness of the ipsilateral lateral rectus, contralateral nystagmus, and normal convergence. Bilateral damage causes internuclear ophthalmoplegia (INO) with no eye adduction.

J. Cranial nerve IX (the glossopharyngeal nerve) (**Fig. A–40**)

   1. The glossopharyngeal nerve leaves the medulla between the olive and the inferior cerebellar peduncle as the most rostral three or four of the rootlets that will form CN IX, X, and XI. The nerve sends off a tympanic branch before exiting the skull through the jugular foramen, where it lies anterior to CN X and XI. The superior and inferior (**petrosal**) glossopharyngeal ganglia are in the jugular foramen.

   2. GSA—sensation from the back of the ear, inner surface of the tympanic membrane, posterior $\frac{1}{3}$ of the tongue, and upper pharynx travels to the superior ganglion to the caudal spinal trigeminal nucleus.

   3. GVA and SVA—the **carotid body and sinus** and taste buds in the **posterior $\frac{1}{3}$ of the tongue**, posterior pharynx, and eustachian tube send fibers to the inferior ganglion (petrosal ganglion) to the caudal nucleus solitarius, which has connections with the reticular formation and hypothalamus.

(a) The taste fibers from the rostral nucleus solitarius ascend in the central tegmental tract to the contralateral thalamic VPM.

(b) Carotid sinus reflex—from the baroreceptor at the carotid bifurcation that senses an increase in blood pressure to CN IX to the nucleus solitarius to the dorsal X nucleus to cause a decrease in blood pressure and heart rate.

(c) Carotid body—a chemoreceptor that detects blood O_2 and CO_2 concentrations. **Hering's nerve** is the branch of CN IX from the carotid body and sinus.

4. GVE—parotid salivation is controlled by fibers from the **inferior salivatory nucleus** to CN IX, to the tympanic nerve (**Jacobson's nerve**) that leaves CN IX before the jugular foramen, goes through the inferior ganglion (that supplies sensation to the tympanic cavity, eustachian tube, and mastoid air cells), through the tympanic plexus, to the **lesser petrosal nerve**, through a small canal lateral to the canal for the greater superficial petrosal nerve back into the cranium, through the foramen ovale, to synapse in the **otic ganglion** (below the foramen ovale and surrounding a branch of V3), and travels with the auriculotemporal nerve (a branch of V3) to the parotid gland.

5. SVE—the rostral nucleus ambiguous innervates the **stylopharyngeus** muscle and part of the superior pharyngeal constrictor.

6. Injury to CN IX—causes decreased gag reflex, decreased sinus reflex, and decreased taste. In isolation, a unilateral injury would be difficult to detect.

7. Glossopharyngeal neuralgia—pain behind the ear or in the mouth often precipitated by swallowing or coughing.

8. Both CN IX and X have two ganglia, but the fibers from CN IX form a single compact root unlike the spread-out fibers from CN X.

K. Cranial nerve X (the vagus nerve)

1. The vagus nerve leaves the medulla between the olive and the inferior cerebellar peduncle as 8 to 10 rootlets that converge into two roots that exit the skull through the jugular foramen. The superior (**jugular**) and inferior (**nodose**) ganglia are just beneath the jugular foramen.

2. GSA—sensation from the ear, external auditory meatus, and external surface of the tympanic membrane travels in the auricular branch (**Arnold's nerve**) and sensation from the posterior fossa dura travels in meningeal branches to the **superior ganglion** of CN X to the spinal trigeminal tract.

(a) Recurrent laryngeal nerve—supplies the vocal cords and subglottis.

(b) Internal laryngeal nerve—supplies the larynx above the vocal folds, pierces the thyrohyoid membrane, and unites with the external laryngeal nerve to form the superior laryngeal nerve.

(c) Fibers from the larynx and pharynx regions go to the inferior ganglion of CN X to the spinal trigeminal tract.

3. GVA and SVA—sensation of the pharynx, larynx, trachea, lungs, heart, esophagus, stomach, and thoracoabdominal viscera down to the splenic flexure, aortic arch baroreceptors, aortic body (chemoreceptor), and taste sensation in the epiglottis travel to the inferior ganglion of CN X to the **tractus solitarius** and the nucleus of the tractus solitarius (fibers from CN VII, IX, and X).

   (a) Rostral part of the nucleus—SVA (gustatory) with input mainly from CN VII and IX.

   (b) Caudal part— mainly GVA from CN X.

   (c) Commissural nucleus—at the obex where both solitary nuclei merge.

   (d) Efferent fibers from the nucleus—to the thalamic VPM, salivary nucleus, the dorsal motor nucleus of CN X, nucleus ambiguous, parabranchial nucleus, hypoglossal nucleus, phrenic nerve nuclei, and thoracic LMN.

   (e) Medullary respiratory center—the nucleus ambiguous, nucleus solitarius, and reticular formation. It responds to vagal input and CO_2 accumulation. The medullary vasomotor center is less well defined.

4. GVE—parasympathetic input arises from the **dorsal motor nucleus of CN X** to the vagus nerve to the thorax and abdomen, where it branches into the right and left gastric nerves that innervate the abdominal viscera up to the splenic flexure. Input to the dorsal motor nucleus of CN X is from the hypothalamus, olfactory system, reticular formation, and the solitary nucleus.

5. SVE—the **nucleus ambiguous** sends fibers to the LMNs for the constrictors of the pharynx and the internal muscles of the larynx. The pharyngeal branch of CN X supplies all the muscles of the pharynx and soft palate except the stylopharyngeus (CN IX) and tensor veli palatini (CN V). These include the superior, middle, and inferior constrictors, levator palati, salpingopharyngeus, palatopharyngeus, and one tongue muscle, the palatoglossus.

   (a) **Superior laryngeal nerve**—divides into the internal and external laryngeal nerves. The external branch supplies the inferior constrictor, cricothyroid, pharyngeal plexus, and superior cardiac nerve.

   (b) **Recurrent laryngeal nerve**—supplies the intrinsic laryngeal muscles except the cricothyroid.

   (c) The nucleus ambiguous also has output to the stylopharyngeus muscle (CN IX) and the trapezius and sternocleidomastoid muscles (CN XI). Rostrally it joins dorsal X and caudally it forms the CN XI nucleus.

6. Unilateral vagal injury—causes hoarseness, dysphagia, dyspnea, uvular deviation to the normal side, ipsilateral decreased cough reflex by decreased sensation, and ipsilateral decreased carotid sinus reflex.

7. Bilateral vagal injury—causes asphyxia, paralysis of the esophagus and stomach with pain and emesis, tachycardia, dysarthria, and dysphagia.

L. Cranial nerve XI (the spinal accessory nerve)

1. SVE—the cranial portion is from the nucleus ambiguous (CN IX, X, and XI) to join with CN X and form the recurrent laryngeal nerve. The spinal portion is from C1-6, exits between the ventral and dorsal roots, ascends posterior to the dentate ligament, enters the foramen magnum, and leaves with the entire CN XI through the jugular foramen. It supplies the sternocleidomastoid and upper trapezius muscles.

M. Cranial nerve XII (the hypoglossal nerve)

1. GSE—the nerve exits the medulla between the inferior olive and the pyramid, travels through the hypoglossal foramen, and innervates all of the intrinsic muscles of the tongue and all but one of the extrinsic muscles of the tongue (the genioglossus, styloglossus, and hypoglossus). The palatoglossus is innervated by CN X.

XVI. BRAIN STEM (FIGS. A–41—A–43)

A. Midbrain—consists of the tectum, tegmentum, and crus cerebri.

1. Level of the superior colliculus—contains the superior colliculus, oculomotor nucleus (V-shaped just ventral to the aqueduct with nerve roots entering the interpeduncular fossa), red nucleus, superior cerebellar peduncle, and substantia nigra (SN).

   (a) Superior colliculus—laminated with alternating gray and white zones. The superficial layers are connected to the visual system and the deep layers are connected to the muscles for head and eye movements.

   (i) Input—by way of the **brachium of the superior colliculus** from the retina (mainly contralateral, unlike the equal representation in the LGB and cortex), cortex (frontal, parietal, temporal, and occipital), brain stem nuclei (parabigeminal nucleus, inferior colliculus, SN, and nucleus cuneatus), and spinal cord.

   (ii) Output—to the parabigeminal nucleus, pulvinar, LGB, PPRF, rostral interstitial nucleus of the MLF (RiMLF), reticular formation, and spinal cord. Unilateral damage causes contralateral visual field neglect, impaired tracking, but no deficit with eye movements.

   (iii) **Stimulation—causes contralateral conjugate deviation**, although there are no direct projections to the extraocular muscles, by (1) stimulating the RiMLF to excite the ipsilateral CN III and (2) stimulating the PPRF to excite the contralateral CN VI and RiMLF.

   (b) Oculomotor nucleus

   (i) Lateral part—has cell columns (all ipsilateral) for the inferior rectus muscle (dorsal), the inferior oblique muscle (intermediate), and the medial rectus muscle (ventral).

   (ii) Medial part—has a cell column for the **contralateral superior rectus muscle**.

   (iii) Central part—has a cell column for both the levator palpebrae superioris muscles and the Edinger-Westphal nuclei.

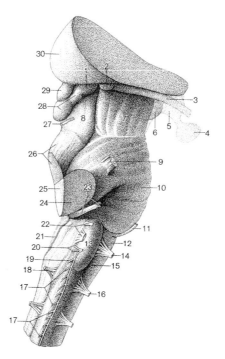

Figure A–41   Brain stem lateral view.

1 Medial geniculate body
2 Lateral geniculate body
3 Optic tract
4 Hypophysis
5 Infundibulum
6 Mamillary body
7, 8 *Cerebral peduncle*
7 Ventral part (crus cerebri)
8 Dorsal part (mesencephalic tegmentum)
9 Trigeminal nerve
10 Pons
11 Abducens nerve
12 Pyramid (medulla oblongata)
13 Olive
14 Hypoglossal nerve
15 Ventrolateral sulcus

16 Ventral root of 1st cervical nerve
17 Spinal roots of accessory nerve
18 Dorsal root of 1st cervical nerve (retracted)
19 Dorsolateral sulcus (medulla oblongata)
20 Cranial roots of accessory nerve and accessory nerve
21 Tenia of 4th ventricle
22 Glossopharyngeal and vagus nerves
23 Facial nerve with nervus intermedius and vestibulocochlear nerve
24 Middle cerebellar peduncle
25 Inferior cerebellar peduncle
26 Superior cerebellar peduncle
27 Trochlear nerve
28 Inferior colliculus and brachium of inferior colliculus
29 Superior colliculus
30 Pulvinar

(iv) Oculomotor rootlets—cross through the red nucleus to enter the interpeduncular fossa. The oculomotor complex has no direct cortical or superior colliculus connections; these all go through reticular formation neurons.

(v) Direct input—bilateral from the medial and ipsilateral superior vestibular nuclei (by way of the MLF), the nucleus of Cajal, the contralateral abducens nucleus, the perihypoglossal nucleus, the RiMLF, and the pretectal olivary nucleus. Also, the flocculus projects to the nucleus prepositus to the ipsilateral oculomotor nucleus for vertical eye movements.

(vi) The PPRF projects directly to the main conjugate horizontal gaze center (abducens nucleus) and the **main conjugate vertical gaze center (the RiMLF)**.

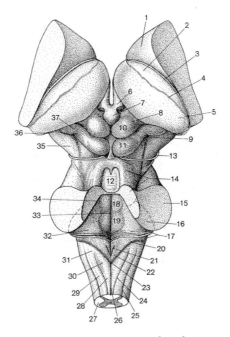

Figure A–42   Brain stem dorsal view.

1 Caudate nucleus
2 Lamina affixa
3 Terminal stria and superior thalamostriate vein in terminal sulcus
4 Tenia choroidea
5 Pulvinar
6 Habenular trigone
7 Pineal body
8–11 *Mesencephalon*
8 Brachium of superior colliculus
9 Brachium of inferior colliculus
10, 11 *Tectum*
10 Superior colliculus
11 Inferior colliculus
12 Superior medullary velum
13 Trochlear nerve
14 Superior cerebellar peduncle
15 Middle cerebellar peduncle
16 Inferior cerebellar peduncle
17 Striae medullares (4th ventricle) and lateral recess (4th ventricle)

18 Medial eminence
19 Facial colliculus
20 Tenia of 4th ventricle
21 Trigone of hypoglossal nerve
22 Trigone of vagus nerve (ala cinerea)
23 Obex
24 Dorsal intermediate sulcus
25 Dorsolateral sulcus (medulla oblongata)
26 Dorsal median sulcus
27 Lateral funiculus
28 Fasciculus gracilis
29 Fasciculus cuneatus
30 Tuberculum gracile
31 Tuberculum cuneatum
32 Vestibular area
33 Median sulcus
34 Sulcus limitans
35 Cerebral peduncle
36 Lateral geniculate body
37 Medial geniculate body

(vii) Direct light reflex—retinal ganglion cells to optic nerve to optic tract to brachium of superior colliculus to **pretectal area** to **posterior commissure** to both oculomotor nuclei to Edinger-Westphal subnucleus to the ciliary ganglion to the pupillary sphincter muscle.

(c) RiMLF—located above the oculomotor nucleus in the MLF at the junction of the midbrain/diencephalon. It is the main center for vertical eye movements (especially downward). It reacts to vestibular and visual stimulation. Input is from the superior vestibular nucleus and PPRF. Output is mainly to the inferior rectus part of the oculomotor complex.

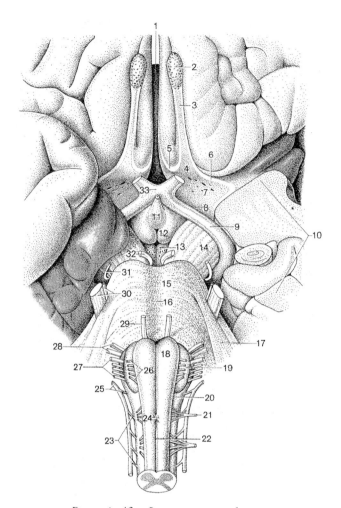

Figure A–43   Brain stem ventral view.

1 Corpus callosum in depth of longitudinal cerebral fissure
2 Olfactory bulb
3 Olfactory tract
4 Olfactory trigone
5 Medial olfactory stria
6 Lateral olfactory stria
7 Anterior perforated substance
8 Diagonal band of *Broca*
9 Optic tract
10 Cut surface of left temporal lobe
11 Infundibulum with hypophysial stalk
12 Mamillary body
13 Interpenducular fossa with interpeduncular perforated substance
14 Ventral part of cerebral peduncle
15 Pons
16 Basilar sulcus
17 Middle cerebellar peduncle

18 Pyramid (medulla oblongata)
19 Olive
20 Ventrolateral sulcus
21 Ventral root of 1st cervical nerve
22 Ventral median fissure
23 Spinal roots of accessory nerve
24 Decussation of pyramid
25 Accessory nerve and cranial roots
26 Root filaments of hypoglossal nerve
27 Glossopharyngeal nerve and root filaments of vagus nerve
28 Facial nerve with nervus intermedius and vestibulocochlear nerve
29 Abducens nerve
30 Motor root and sensory root of trigeminal nerve
31 Trochlear nerve
32 Oculomotor nerve
33 Optic chiasma

(d) Accessory oculomotor nuclei

    (i)   Interstitial nucleus of Cajal—located along the MLF in the rostral midbrain. Input is from the superior and medial vestibular nuclei, pretectum, frontal eye fields, and the fastigial nuclei. Output is to the ipsilateral medial vestibular nucleus and spinal cord, both trochlear nuclei, and the contralateral oculomotor nuclei (crossing in the posterior commissure) although not to the medial rectus part. It functions with vertical eye movements, pursuit, head movements, and posture.

    (ii)   Darkschevich's nucleus—located dorsolateral to the oculomotor nucleus and output is to the nucleus of the posterior commissure.

    (iii)   Nucleus of the posterior commissure—connections with the pretectal area and posterior thalamic nuclei.

(e) Pretectal region—located just rostral to the superior colliculus at the posterior commissure. Nuclei are involved with pupillary light reflexes.

(f) Posterior commissure—posterior to the aqueduct, at the junction of the midbrain/diencephalon. It is involved with the light reflex and contains fibers from the pretectal nuclei, nucleus of the posterior commissure, interstitial nuclei, and Darkschevich's nucleus.

(g) Subcommissural organ—modified ependymal cells in the aqueduct below the posterior commissure. It has no blood brain barrier.

2. Level of the inferior colliculus—the inferior colliculus is responsible for the tonotopic organization of auditory information and projects by way of the brachium of the inferior colliculus to the MGB.

    (a) **Parabigeminal area**—ventrolateral to the inferior colliculus, with connections to the superior colliculus. It is involved with the visual system.

    (b) Trochlear nucleus roots—cross in the superior medullary velum, emerge on the contralateral side under the inferior colliculus, travel between the PCA and SCA with the oculomotor nerve, and enter the cavernous sinus.

    (c) **Periaqueductal gray**—contains the mesencephalic nucleus of V, the locus ceruleus, dorsal nucleus of the raphe (sends 5-HT and CCK to the SN and putamen), ventral and dorsal tegmental nuclei, and the median nucleus of the raphe (forms the mesolimbic system with output to the brain stem reticular formation, hypothalamus, septal area, entorhinal cortex, hippocampus, cerebellum, locus ceruleus, and raphe nucleus of the pons and medulla).

        (i)   Function—it is involved with central **analgesia**, vocalization, control of reproductive behavior, aggressive behavior, and upward gaze.

        (ii)   Connections—to the hypothalamus, reticular formation, spinal cord, locus ceruleus, and raphe nucleus.

    (d) **Interpeduncular nucleus**—located just dorsal to the interpeduncular fossa. Input is from the habenular nucleus by way of the fasciculus retroflexus and there is **diffuse output with cholinergic fibers** to various parts of the CNS.

3. Midbrain tegmentum—contains the reticular formation, red nucleus, oculomotor and trochlear nuclei, etc.

   (a) Red nucleus—located in the reticular formation. Fibers of the oculomotor nerve and the superior cerebellar peduncle pass through it.

      (i) Input—from (1) the deep cerebellar nuclei—rostral $\frac{1}{3}$ from the **dentate nuclei** and caudal $\frac{2}{3}$ from the **interposed nuclei**; fibers exit the cerebellum by way of the superior peduncle and cross to the contralateral side in the midbrain to reach the red nucleus, and (2) the **cerebral cortex**—from the precentral, premotor, supplementary motor, and motor cortices.

      (ii) Output—to (1) the contralateral cervical and lumbar spine by way of the **rubrospinal tract**, (2) the contralateral interposed nuclei, facial nucleus, medulla, and spinal cord by way of the crossed ventral tegmental tract, and (3) the ipsilateral inferior olivary nucleus by way of the uncrossed **central tegmental tract**.

      (iii) There are no direct connections to the thalamus. **Stimulation elicits increased tone in the contralateral flexors and decreased in the contralateral extensors.** It functions to maintain flexor muscle tone. Stimulation of the interposed nucleus elicits increased ipsilateral flexion.

   (b) Midbrain reticular formation.

   (c) **Pedunculopontine nucleus**—located in the lateral tegmentum ventral to the inferior colliculus. Input is from the cortex, mGP, and SNpr. Output is to the thalamus and SNpc. It is one of the **major sources of ACh output**. It is involved with control of locomotion. Stimulation causes walking movements.

4. Substantia nigra (SN)—located between the crus cerebri and midbrain tegmentum.

   (a) SNpc—contains large cells and uses **dopamine (DA)** and CCK as neurotransmitters.

   (b) SNpr—has fewer cells, is ventral to the SNpc and therefore closer to the crus cerebri, and uses GABA and 5-HT.

   (c) Input—from the caudate and putamen and lateral (GP to the SNpr [GABA]), subthalamus, dorsal raphe nucleus (5-HT and CCK), and the pedunculopontine nucleus (ACh). There is also input with enkephalin and substance P (the highest concentration in the brain).

   (d) Output—(1) SNpc with DA to the striatum as a closed loop, (2) SNpr to the VA and MD thalamus, (3) SNpr to the superior colliculus (initiates eye movements) and the pedunculopontine nucleus. The striatum loop sends GABA, substance P, and enkephalin to the SNpr to the SNpc sending DA back to the striatum.

5. Crus cerebri—middle $\frac{2}{3}$ is corticospinal and corticobulbar tracts with lower extremities lateral. The extreme medial and lateral ends are corticopontine with frontopontine medial and parieto-temporo-occipitopontine laterally. One million of the 20 million fibers are corticospinal.

B. Pons

1. Reticular formation—located in the pons and medulla and has four zones.

    (a) Median zone—contains the raphe nuclei. The dorsal and median raphe nuclei send the ventral tegmental tract to the median forebrain bundle to the hypothalamus, striatum, thalamus, amygdala, hippocampus, cortex, and olfactory bulb.

    (b) Paramedian zone—input from cortex and so on and output to cerebellum.

    (c) Medial zone—the effector zone with ascending and descending fibers.

    (d) Lateral zone—the sensory zone with output to the effector zone.

    (e) Stimulation—induces reflexes and cortically induced movements.

    (f) Pontine reticular formation—sends crossed reticulospinal fibers to the LMN of the spinal cord and the central tegmental tract to the thalamic intralaminar nuclei for arousal. The reticular formation is involved with muscle tone (reticulospinal tract), sensory transmission, wakefulness (central tegmental tract), respiration, and blood pressure.

    (g) The bulbar pressor area is the main control and the depressor area is in the rostral medulla/caudal pons.

    (h) **Ascending reticular activating system (ARAS)**—involved with cortical arousal. The main ascending pathway is the central tegmental tract to the rostral intralaminar thalamic nuclei.

2. The isthmus rhombencephali between the cerebellum and midbrain has the superior medullary velum with the decussating trochlear nerves over the roof of the fourth ventricle. The parabranchial nuclei are adjacent to the superior cerebellar peduncles.

3. **Locus ceruleus**—pigmented (melanin) and uses **norepinephrine (NE)** as the neurotransmitter with wide projections. It controls cortical activation and paradoxical (REM) sleep.

C. Medulla—the olivary level of the medulla

1. Floor of the fourth ventricle—three eminences (medial to lateral): (1) the hypoglossal eminence over the CN XII nucleus, (2) the intermediate eminence over CN X (medially is the dorsal motor nucleus of CN X and laterally is the solitary nucleus), and (3) the lateral eminence over the area vestibularis. The sulcus limitans separates the efferent and afferent (lateral) fibers. The roof is the tela choroidea and the choroid plexus lies in the inferior medullary velum.

2. **Inferior olivary complex**—principal olivary nucleus sends efferent fibers to the cerebellum (especially hemispheres); the medial and dorsal accessory olivary nuclei send fibers to the vermis. The olivocerebellar fibers cross to the inferior cerebellar peduncles (they make up most of the peduncle) and become climbing fibers to reach Purkinje's cells. The complex also sends descending fibers.

3. Medullary reticular formation—afferent fibers are from the cortex, deep cerebellar nuclei, and cranial nerves. Output is from the gigantocellular reticular nucleus to (1) central tegmental tract

crossed to the intralaminar thalamic nuclei for arousal and also from the midbrain to the olive, and (2) reticulospinal tract (rostral fibers stimulate and caudal fibers inhibit LMNs).

4. **Raphe nuclei**—extend from the midbrain to the medulla. Their neurotransmitters include **serotonin**, CCK, and enkephalin. They provide endogenous analgesia by way of the substantia gelatinosa and control deep sleep, mood, and aggression. The nucleus magnus projects to layers 1 and 2 in the spinal cord to inhibit pain. If there is less firing, there is less arousal, but destruction causes insomnia.

5. Tracts—the medial lemniscus (ML), spinothalamic tracts (the anterior and lateral tracts merge and branch to the reticular formation), dorsal spinocerebellar tract to the inferior peduncle, ventral spinocerebellar tract to the superior cerebellar peduncle, the MLF, rubrospinal, rubrobulbar, and vestibulospinal tracts.

6. Inferior cerebellar peduncles—carry fibers from the spinal cord and medulla to the cerebellum. Most are crossed olivocerebellar fibers, uncrossed dorsal spinocerebellar fibers, uncrossed fibers from the lateral vestibular nuclei, and fibers from the paramedian reticular nuclei, accessory cuneate nuclei, arcuate nuclei, and perihypoglossal nuclei.

D. Spinomedullary junction

1. Internal changes—decussation of the pyramids, termination of the fasciculi gracilus and cuneatus, replacement of the Lissauer's zone by the spinal trigeminal tract, replacement of the spinal gray by the reticular formation, and the cranial nerve nuclei.

2. Corticospinal decussation—anterior corticospinal tract travels in the anterior fasciculus and is mostly uncrossed. The lateral corticospinal tract travels in the dorsolateral fasciculus and is mostly crossed.

3. Decussation of the medial lemniscus—dorsal root ganglion (DRG) to the posterior column fibers to the nucleus gracilus (lower extremities) and cuneatus (upper extremities) cross as the **internal arcuate fibers** to the **medial lemniscus** to the VPL to the sensory cortex. There is somatotopic organization with touch and kinesthetic fibers intermingled.

    (a) **Accessory cuneate nucleus**—lateral and rostral to the cuneate nucleus. It serves a similar function to Clarke's column in the thorax to send fibers that are the UE equivalent of the posterior spinocerebellar tract.

    (b) The UE muscle spindles, Golgi's tendon organs, and cutaneous afferent fibers go to the primary spinal ganglion to the second neurons in the accessory cuneate nucleus to the cuneocerebellar fibers to the inferior cerebellar peduncle.

4. The spinal trigeminal tract and nucleus with input from the CNs V, VII, IX, and X.

5. Reticular formation—fibers from the red nucleus and spinothalamic tract to the reticular nuclei to the inferior peduncles and up as mossy fibers. The cortex to the arcuate nuclei (anterior to the pyramids) to the stria medullaris (floor of the fourth ventricle) to the cerebellum.

6. **Area postrema**—in the floor of the fourth ventricle above the obex. It is a chemoreceptor sensitive to apomorphine and digitalis with afferent fibers from the spinal cord and nucleus solitarius.

E. Associations (**Table A–2**)

TABLE A–2. ASSOCIATIONS

Brain stem	Artery	Cranial nerves	Cerebellar peduncle	Cerebellar surface
Midbrain	SCA	Under CN III and IV and above CN V	Superior	Tentorial
Pons	AICA	Passes CN VI, VII, and VIII	Middle	Petrosal
Medulla	PICA	Passes CN XII, IX, X, and XI	Inferior	Suboccipital

XVII. SPINE AND SPINAL CORD

A. General information

1. Spinal cord **(Figs. A–44—A–50)**—extends from the foramen magnum to L1/2 in the adult. The cervical and lumbar enlargements contain the LMNs for the upper and lower extremities, respectively. The spinal cord tapers to a distal end called the conus medullaris. The long nerve roots extending past the conus medullaris form the cauda equina. The filum terminale consists of pia from the conus medullaris, rests of ependymal cells, glia, and fat that extend through the thecal sac to its end at S2 and together with the dura form the coccygeal ligament that attaches to the posterior coccyx.

2. There are 31 pairs of spinal nerves and spinal segments that have paired ventral and dorsal roots (8 cervical, 12 thoracic, 5 lumbar, 5 sacral, and 1 coccygeal) **(Figs A–51 and A–52)**. At 3 months' gestation, the spinal cord extends to the end of the spinal canal. At birth, the conus is at L3, and in the adult it is at L1/2.

3. Nerve roots—exit through the intervertebral foramen. The C1 root exits between the occiput and the atlas. The cervical roots exit above their respective pedicles, except for the C8 root that exits between C7 and T1. All of the other roots exit under their respective pedicles. There is no dorsal root for C1, so there is no C1 sensory dermatome.

4. In the posterior nerve roots, the pain and temmperature fibers are lateral and the posterior column fibers are medial.

5. Dorsal root ganglion (DRG)—The primary cell bodies for the sensory pathways are located in the dorsal root (spinal) ganglia that reside in the spinal intervertebral foramen. There are no synapses here because the pseudo-unipolar axon divides in a "T"–line fusion with a peripheral branch connected to a sensory receptor, and a central branch entering via the dorsal spinal root to the spinal cord.

6. The anterior median fissure extends deeply to near the gray commissure. The posterior median sulcus extends down to the posterior median septum. There are two posterolateral sulci near the dorsal root entry zones (DREZ). The posterior intermediate sulci separate the fasciculus gracilius from the fasciculus cuneatus.

7. Three paired funiculi:

    (a) Anterior funiculus—extends from the anterior median fissure to the ventral root.

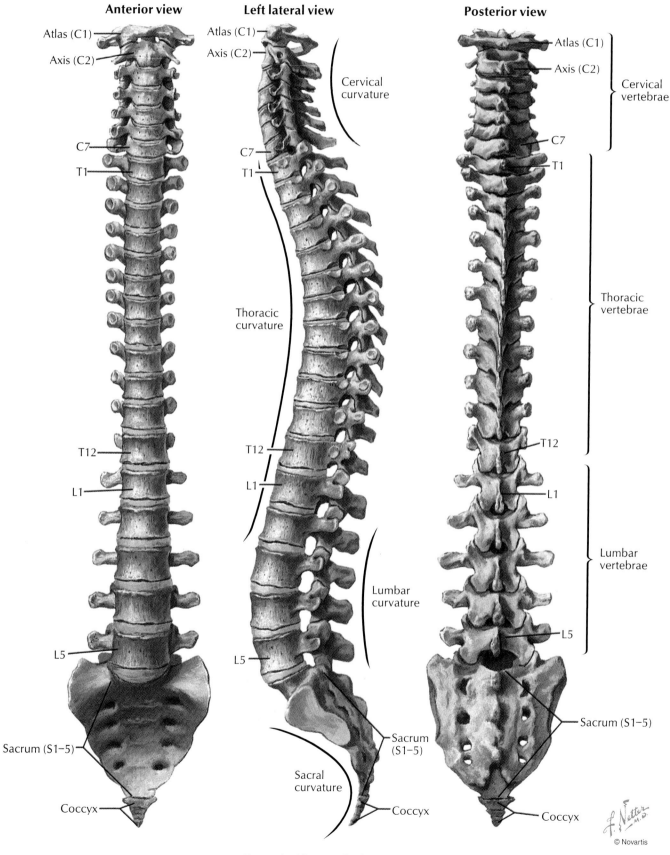

Anterior view

Atlas (C1)
Axis (C2)

C7
T1

T12

L1

L5

Sacrum (S1–5)

Coccyx

Left lateral view

Atlas (C1)
Axis (C2)

Cervical
curvature

C7
T1

Thoracic
curvature

T12

L1

L5

Lumbar
curvature

Sacrum
(S1–5)

Sacral
curvature

Coccyx

Posterior view

Atlas (C1)
Axis (C2)

Cervical
vertebrae

C7
T1

Thoracic
vertebrae

T12

L1

Lumbar
vertebrae

L5

Sacrum (S1–5)

Coccyx

© Novartis

Figure A–44   Vertebral column.

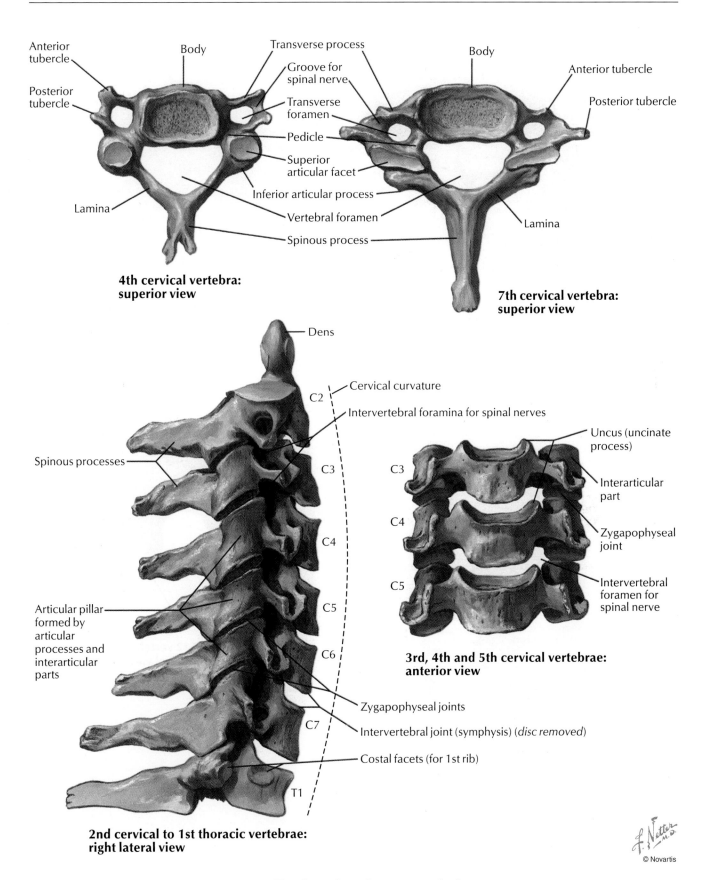

Anterior tubercle

Body

Transverse process

Groove for spinal nerve

Transverse foramen

Pedicle

Superior articular facet

Inferior articular process

Vertebral foramen

Spinous process

Posterior tubercle

Lamina

4th cervical vertebra: superior view

Body

Anterior tubercle

Posterior tubercle

Lamina

7th cervical vertebra: superior view

Dens

Cervical curvature

C2

Intervertebral foramina for spinal nerves

C3

Spinous processes

C4

Articular pillar formed by articular processes and interarticular parts

C5

C6

Zygapophyseal joints

C7

Intervertebral joint (symphysis) (*disc removed*)

Costal facets (for 1st rib)

T1

2nd cervical to 1st thoracic vertebrae: right lateral view

Uncus (uncinate process)

C3

Interarticular part

C4

Zygapophyseal joint

C5

Intervertebral foramen for spinal nerve

3rd, 4th and 5th cervical vertebrae: anterior view

© Novartis

Figure A–45　Cervical vertebrae, uncovertebral joint.

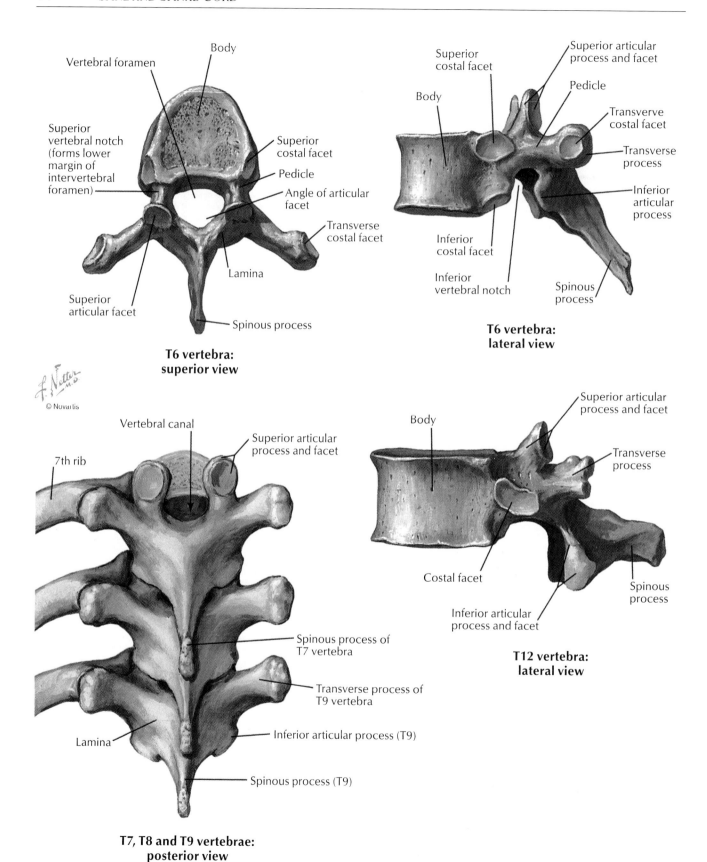

Body

Vertebral foramen

Superior
vertebral notch
(forms lower
margin of
intervertebral
foramen)

Superior
costal facet

Pedicle

Angle of articular
facet

Transverse
costal facet

Lamina

Superior
articular facet

Spinous process

**T6 vertebra:
superior view**

Superior
costal facet

Body

Superior articular
process and facet

Pedicle

Transverve
costal facet

Transverse
process

Inferior
articular
process

Inferior
costal facet

Inferior
vertebral notch

Spinous
process

**T6 vertebra:
lateral view**

Vertebral canal

Superior articular
process and facet

7th rib

Spinous process of
T7 vertebra

Transverse process of
T9 vertebra

Inferior articular process (T9)

Lamina

Spinous process (T9)

**T7, T8 and T9 vertebrae:
posterior view**

Body

Superior articular
process and facet

Transverse
process

Inferior articular
process and facet

Costal facet

Spinous
process

**T12 vertebra:
lateral view**

Figure A–46   Thoracic vertebrae.

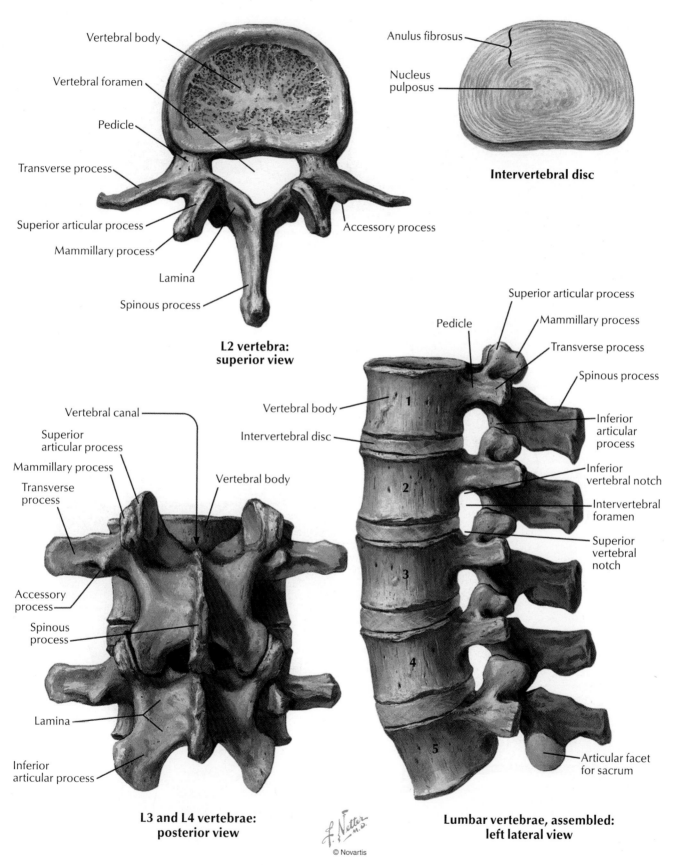

L2 vertebra:
superior view

Intervertebral disc

L3 and L4 vertebrae:
posterior view

Lumbar vertebrae, assembled:
left lateral view

Figure A—47   Lumbar vertebrae.

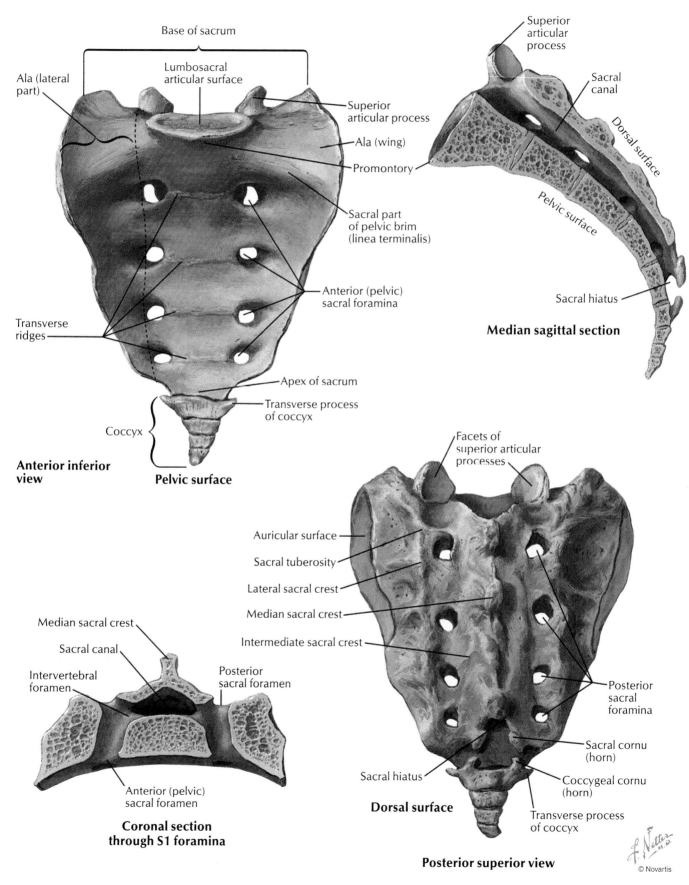

Base of sacrum

Ala (lateral part)

Lumbosacral articular surface

Superior articular process

Ala (wing)

Promontory

Sacral part of pelvic brim (linea terminalis)

Anterior (pelvic) sacral foramina

Transverse ridges

Apex of sacrum

Transverse process of coccyx

Coccyx

Anterior inferior view

Pelvic surface

Superior articular process

Sacral canal

Dorsal surface

Pelvic surface

Sacral hiatus

Median sagittal section

Facets of superior articular processes

Auricular surface

Sacral tuberosity

Lateral sacral crest

Median sacral crest

Intermediate sacral crest

Posterior sacral foramina

Sacral cornu (horn)

Coccygeal cornu (horn)

Sacral hiatus

Transverse process of coccyx

Dorsal surface

Posterior superior view

Median sacral crest

Sacral canal

Intervertebral foramen

Posterior sacral foramen

Anterior (pelvic) sacral foramen

Coronal section through S1 foramina

© Novartis

Figure A–48   Sacrum and coccyx.

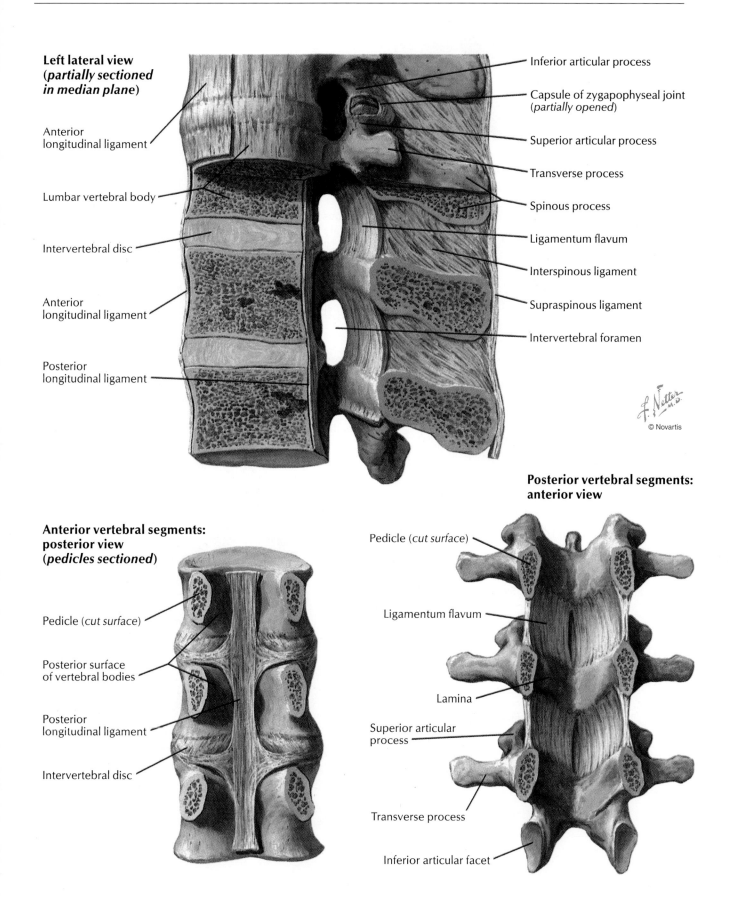

Left lateral view (*partially sectioned in median plane*)

Anterior longitudinal ligament

Lumbar vertebral body

Intervertebral disc

Anterior longitudinal ligament

Posterior longitudinal ligament

Inferior articular process

Capsule of zygapophyseal joint (*partially opened*)

Superior articular process

Transverse process

Spinous process

Ligamentum flavum

Interspinous ligament

Supraspinous ligament

Intervertebral foramen

Posterior vertebral segments: anterior view

Pedicle (*cut surface*)

Ligamentum flavum

Lamina

Superior articular process

Transverse process

Inferior articular facet

Anterior vertebral segments: posterior view (*pedicles sectioned*)

Pedicle (*cut surface*)

Posterior surface of vertebral bodies

Posterior longitudinal ligament

Intervertebral disc

Figure A–49   Vertebral ligaments, lumbar region.

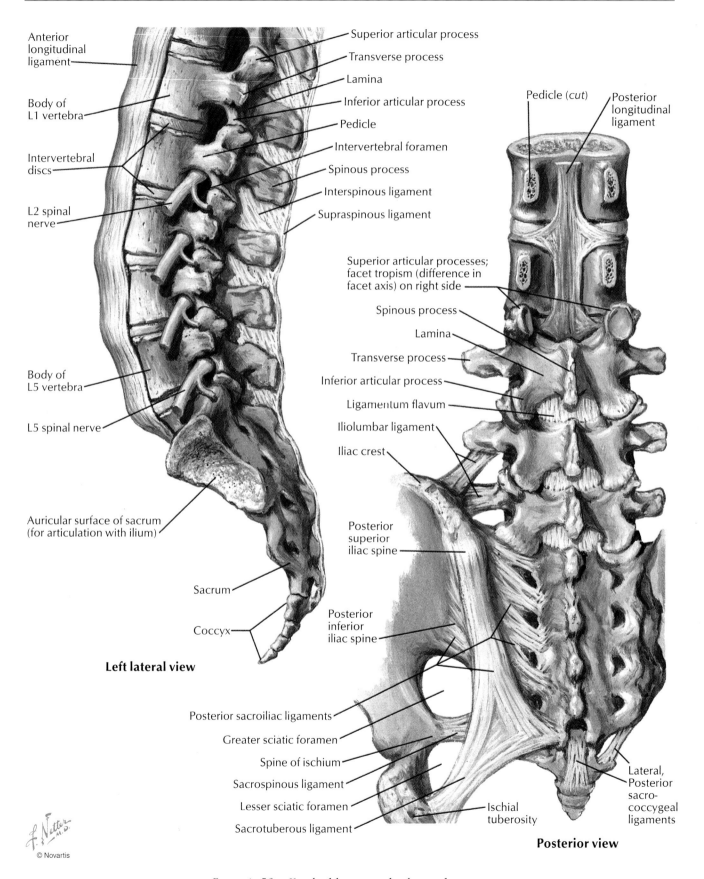

Anterior longitudinal ligament

Body of L1 vertebra

Intervertebral discs

L2 spinal nerve

Body of L5 vertebra

L5 spinal nerve

Auricular surface of sacrum (for articulation with ilium)

Sacrum

Coccyx

Left lateral view

Superior articular process

Transverse process

Lamina

Inferior articular process

Pedicle

Intervertebral foramen

Spinous process

Interspinous ligament

Supraspinous ligament

Pedicle (*cut*)

Posterior longitudinal ligament

Superior articular processes; facet tropism (difference in facet axis) on right side

Spinous process

Lamina

Transverse process

Inferior articular process

Ligamentum flavum

Iliolumbar ligament

Iliac crest

Posterior superior iliac spine

Posterior inferior iliac spine

Posterior sacroiliac ligaments

Greater sciatic foramen

Spine of ischium

Sacrospinous ligament

Lesser sciatic foramen

Sacrotuberous ligament

Ischial tuberosity

Lateral, Posterior sacro-coccygeal ligaments

Posterior view

Figure A–50   Vertebral ligaments, lumbosacral region.

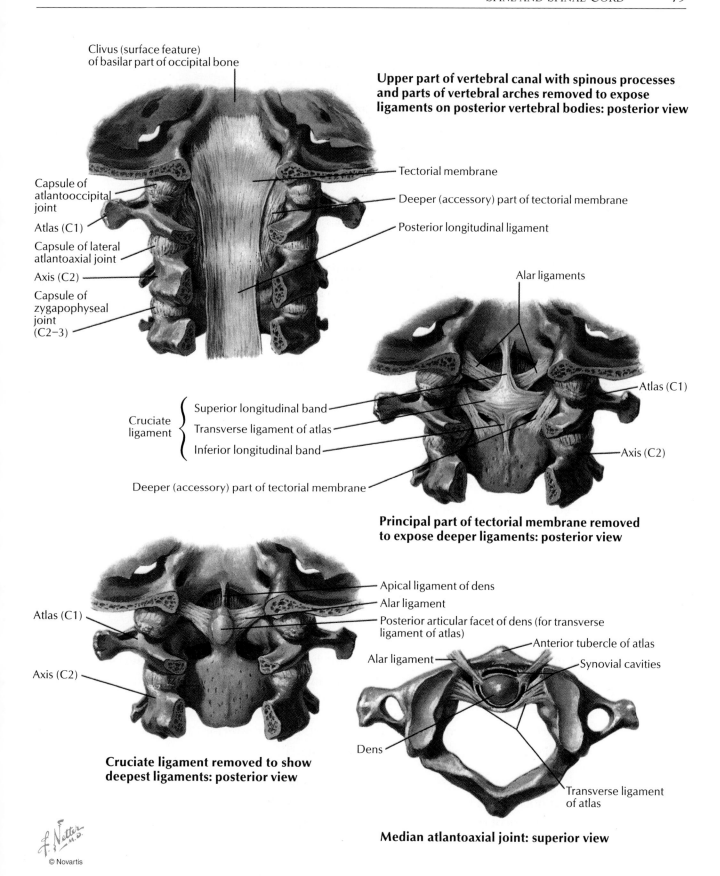

Clivus (surface feature) of basilar part of occipital bone

Upper part of vertebral canal with spinous processes and parts of vertebral arches removed to expose ligaments on posterior vertebral bodies: posterior view

Tectorial membrane

Deeper (accessory) part of tectorial membrane

Posterior longitudinal ligament

Capsule of atlantooccipital joint

Atlas (C1)

Capsule of lateral atlantoaxial joint

Axis (C2)

Capsule of zygapophyseal joint (C2–3)

Alar ligaments

Atlas (C1)

Axis (C2)

Cruciate ligament
Superior longitudinal band
Transverse ligament of atlas
Inferior longitudinal band

Deeper (accessory) part of tectorial membrane

Principal part of tectorial membrane removed to expose deeper ligaments: posterior view

Apical ligament of dens

Alar ligament

Posterior articular facet of dens (for transverse ligament of atlas)

Alar ligament

Anterior tubercle of atlas

Synovial cavities

Dens

Transverse ligament of atlas

Atlas (C1)

Axis (C2)

Cruciate ligament removed to show deepest ligaments: posterior view

Median atlantoaxial joint: superior view

© Novartis

Figure A–51   Craniocervical ligaments.

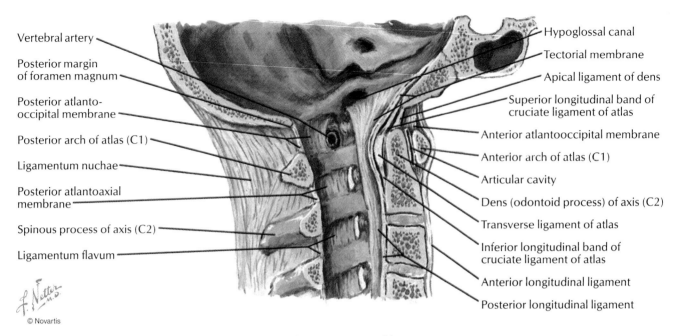

Vertebral artery

Posterior margin
of foramen magnum

Posterior atlanto-
occipital membrane

Posterior arch of atlas (C1)

Ligamentum nuchae

Posterior atlantoaxial
membrane

Spinous process of axis (C2)

Ligamentum flavum

© Novartis

Hypoglossal canal

Tectorial membrane

Apical ligament of dens

Superior longitudinal band of
cruciate ligament of atlas

Anterior atlantooccipital membrane

Anterior arch of atlas (C1)

Articular cavity

Dens (odontoid process) of axis (C2)

Transverse ligament of atlas

Inferior longitudinal band of
cruciate ligament of atlas

Anterior longitudinal ligament

Posterior longitudinal ligament

Figure A–52   Craniocervical ligaments.

(b) Lateral funiculus—between the ventral roots and dorsal roots.

(c) Posterior funiculi—extends from the posterior horn to the posterior median septum, is divided in the upper thoracic and cervical cord by a posterior intermediate septum, is the largest funiculus, and is mainly composed of ascending fibers from the dorsal root ganglia.

(d) Anterior and lateral funiculi—contain ascending fibers from the spinal gray and descending fibers from the brain stem and cortex.

8. Central gray—butterfly shaped. The posterior horns extend almost to the surface, whereas the anterior horns only extend out a short distance. The lateral horn is noted in the thoracic cord. The gray commissure is around the central canal.

9. Cervical cord—oval shaped, being wider than tall. In the posterior funiculi the fasciculus gracilis is medial and the fasciculus cuneatus is lateral.

10. Thoracic cord—contains less gray matter. There is no fasciculus cuneatus at the lower levels. The lateral horn contains the intermediolateral cell column. The dorsal nucleus of Clarke is located at the base of the dorsal horn and extends throughout the thoracic cord but is especially large at T10-L2.

11. Lumbar cord—nearly circular, contains much gray matter, and has less white matter than the cervical cord. The sacral cord is similar to the lumbar cord.

B. Rexed's laminae

   1. Ten layers determined by Rexed, but there is no layer VI between T4-L2.

   2. Layer I—the posteromarginal nucleus (**marginal zone**) caps the surface of the dorsal horn. Input is from DRG and layer II. The DRG axons ascend or descend over layer I in Lissauer's tract before synapsing. Layer I is mainly involved with pain and temperature (**fast pain, Aδ**) that travels in the contralateral spinothalamic tract. Neurotransmitters are substance P, enkephalin, 5-HT, and somatostatin.

   3. Layer II—the **substantia gelatinosa**. Input is from the posterior columns and the dorsolateral and lateral funiculi, with **C fibers (slow pain)**. It modulates sensation by influencing layers III and IV, but there are no ascending pathways. The neurotransmitter is substance P.

   4. Layers I and II—have large amounts of **substance P and opiate receptors**. Output is to the ventral and lateral horns for reflexes and rostrally for sensory transmission.

   5. Layers III and IV—the **nucleus proprius**. Interneurons that convey low intensity stimuli to the thalamus.

   6. Layer V—unknown function.

   7. Layer VI—input is group 1 muscle afferents to the medial zone and descending spinal pathways to the lateral zone.

   8. Layer VII—**the zona intermedia**. It lies between the anterior and posterior horns and includes the lateral horns. The **dorsal nucleus of Clarke** extends from C8-L2 and sends fibers to the ipsilateral dorsal spinocerebellar tract (the contralateral ventral spinocerebellar tract comes from cells in layers V and VI). The **intermediolateral cell column** sends sympathetic fibers out with the ventral roots by way of the white rami communicantes. The parasympathetic output is from the sacral area (S2-4) by way of the pelvic nerves. The intermediomedial cell column is the medial part of layer VII and extends the entire length of the cord with visceral input. The central cervical nucleus is from C1-4 and sends crossed fibers to the cerebellum and inferior vestibular nucleus.

   9. Layer VIII—at the base of the anterior horn.

10. Layer IX—contains the **alpha and gamma motor neurons**. The medial nuclear group controls the axial muscles. The lateral nuclear group controls the limb's appendicular muscles. The ventral group controls extensors, and the dorsal group controls flexors.

11. Layer X—unknown.

12. Dorsal root afferents—the medial bundle has large myelinated fibers to the posterior columns or medial posterior horn from the encapsulated receptors such as the Golgi tendon organs, muscle spindles, Pacinian corpuscles, Meissner's corpuscles, and so on. The **lateral bundle is thinner and contains thinly or nonmyelinated fibers** conveying crude touch, pain, and temperature from free nerve endings. There are collateral fibers for reflexes. The thick fibers pass through or around layer II to end on layers III and IV, or they may end on Clarke's column. The primary neurotransmitter in the spinal and cranial sensory ganglia is glutamate.

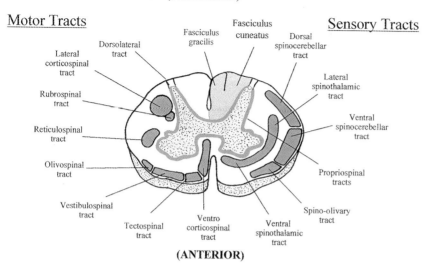

(POSTERIOR)

Motor Tracts

Sensory Tracts

Lateral corticospinal tract

Dorsolateral tract

Fasciculus gracilis

Fasciculus cuneatus

Dorsal spinocerebellar tract

Rubrospinal tract

Lateral spinothalamic tract

Reticulospinal tract

Ventral spinocerebellar tract

Olivospinal tract

Propriospinal tracts

Vestibulospinal tract

Spino-olivary tract

Tectospinal tract

Ventro corticospinal tract

Ventral spinothalamic tract

(ANTERIOR)

Figure A–53   Spinal cord pathways.

C. Spinal cord tracts (**Figs. A–53 and A–54**)

1. Ascending tracts

    (a) Posterior columns—convey fine touch, vibration, and proprioception. The lower extremity fibers are medial. The posterior intermediate septum starts at T6 and divides the fasciculi gracilis and cuneatus. Most lower extremity group I afferent fibers (Ia from muscle spindles and Ib from Golgi tendon organs) go to Clarke's column and the dorsal spinocerebellar tract, not the fasciculus gracilis and posterior columns. The descending fibers in the posterior column go to layer VI.

    (b) Anterior spinothalamic tract—conveys mainly light touch. Fibers originate from layers I, IV, and V and most cross in the anterior commissure, but 10% remain ipsilateral. Fibers terminate in the reticular formation, periaqueductal gray, intralaminar thalamic nuclei, and the thalamic VPL. The lower extremity fibers are lateral.

    (c) Lateral spinothalamic tract—conveys pain and temperature. Fibers are from layers I, IV, and V and cross to ascend in the contralateral lateral spinothalamic tract to the reticular formation and thalamic VPL.

    (d) Spinotectal tract—may convey pain stimuli. Fibers are from layers I and V, cross to the anterolateral spinal cord, and ascend to the superior colliculi and periaqueductal gray.

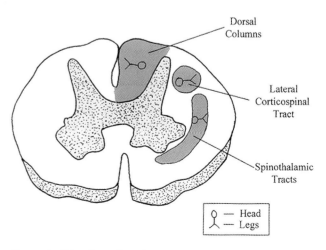

Dorsal Columns

Lateral Corticospinal Tract

Spinothalamic Tracts

Q — Head
X — Legs

Figure A–54   Spinal cord somatotopic organization.

(e) Dorsal spinocerebellar tract—conveys touch, pressure, and proprioception from the lower extremities. Type Ia and b and II fibers from the Golgi tendon organs and muscle spindles go to Clarke's nucleus (C8-L3) to the ipsilateral dorsal spinocerebellar tract in the posterolateral spinal cord to the inferior cerebellar peduncle to the cerebellar vermis.

(f) Ventral spinocerebellar tract—conveys lower extremity posture and coordination information from the Golgi tendon organs by means of Ib fibers to layers V, VI, and VII to a nucleus (LI-coccyx) and samples efference copies of the motor command reaching the alpha motor neurons. Fibers are bilateral but mainly crossed to the contralateral ventral spinocerebellar tract to the superior cerebellar peduncle and cross again to the anterior vermis. Most of the path is contralateral. There is no loss of touch or proprioception noted with disruption of this path because there is no conscious processing of this information.

(g) Cuneocerebellar tract—conveys touch, pressure, and proprioception from the upper extremities (upper extremity equivalent of the dorsal spinocerebellar tract). Ia and b fibers travel in the fasciculus cuneatus to the accessory cuneate nucleus in the medulla to the cuneocerebellar tract up the inferior peduncle to lobule 5 of the cerebellum.

(h) Rostral spinocerebellar tract—the UE equivalent of the ventral spinocerebellar tract providing efference copies, ipsilateral, and enters the inferior peduncle.

(i) Spino-olivary tract—conveys cutaneous and group Ib receptor impulses from the DRG to the posterior columns to the nuclei cuneatus and gracilus to the accessory olivary nucleus and crosses to the contralateral anterior lobe of the cerebellum. There are also fibers from the DRG that cross and travel in the anterior spinal cord to the dorsal and medial accessory olivary nucleus.

(j) Spinoreticular tract—modulates motor, sensory, behavior, and awareness. Impulses travel in the anterolateral spinal cord ipsilaterally to the reticular formation in the medulla, bilaterally to the pons, and bilaterally to the midbrain.

2. Descending tracts

(a) Corticospinal tract—conveys voluntary skilled movements. Fibers are from Betz's cells (only **3%** of fibers) in layer 5 of the motor cortex (area 4, **30%** of fibers), premotor (area 6, **30%** of fibers), and postcentral (areas 3, 1, and 2) and parietal (area 5) cortex (**40%** of fibers from the parietal lobe). The fibers go through the pyramid (1 million fibers, **60% myelinated**) to the medulla/spinal cord junction.

(i) Lateral corticospinal tract—90% of the fibers, almost all are crossed, travels in the posterolateral funiculus, and enters the intermediate gray to laminas IV, V, VI, and VII. A few to the anterior horns in lamina 9.

(ii) Anterior corticospinal tract—10% of the fibers, ipsilateral but crosses in the anterior white commissure to lamina VII.

(iii) Anterolateral corticospinal tract—Ipsilateral, to the posterior horn and intermediate gray. **Glutamate and aspartate** are the neurotransmitters.

(b) Tectospinal tract—involved with **reflex posture movements** in response to visual and possibly auditory stimuli. Fibers from the **superior colliculi** cross in the midbrain to join the MLF at the medulla and travel in the anterior funiculus to the cervical levels C1-4. They synapse in laminas VI, VII, and VIII and have more direct connections to the anterior motor neurons than the corticospinal tracts.

(c) Rubrospinal tract—involved with maintenance of **flexor tone.** Fibers from the red nuclei cross in the ventral tegmentum; travel anteriorly and partially intermingle with the corticospinal tract; descend to laminas V, VI, and VII over the entire length of the cord. The red nucleus has input from both cerebral cortices and the contralateral cerebellar interposed nuclei by way of the superior peduncle. There is somatotopic organization from the cortex to the spinal cord. Stimulation of the red nucleus causes contralateral flexion and inhibits extension.

(d) Vestibulospinal tract—involved with maintenance of **extensor tone.** Fibers from the lateral vestibular nucleus travel ipsilaterally the length of the spinal cord in the anterior part of the lateral funiculus to laminas VII, VIII, and IX, and directly to the alpha and gamma motor neurons and interneurons. There is somatotopic organization, and stimulation causes extension.

(e) Pontine reticulospinal tract—involved with maintenance of **extensor tone** (antigravity muscles) in the axial more than limb muscles, especially the neck. Fibers from the medial pons travel ipsilaterally in the medial anterior funiculus near the MLF and go the entire length of the cord to laminas VII and VIII. Fibers are not somatotopic.

(f) Medullary reticulospinal tract—involved with **inhibition of extensor tone.** Fibers from the medial reticular formation of the medulla (especially the nucleus reticularis gigantocellularis) travel bilaterally in the anterior part of the lateral funiculus the length of the cord to lamina VII. Fibers are not somatotopic. The lateral tegmental system conveys impulses from the reticular formation to the spinal cord for sympathetic control. This system has much cortical input and influences voluntary movement, muscle tone, respiration, pressor/depressor function, and regulation of sensory impulses. The nucleus raphe magnus sends fibers bilaterally in the dorsolateral funiculus to laminas I, II, and V in the cervical enlargement.

(g) Medial longitudinal fasciculus (MLF)—involved with head, neck, and eye movements. Fibers travel in the posterior part of the anterior funiculus with input from the medial and inferior vestibular nuclei, pontine reticular formation, superior colliculus, and interstitial nucleus of Cajal mainly to the cervical segments in laminas VII and VIII.

(h) Descending autonomic pathways—travel from the hypothalamus, Edinger-Westphal nucleus, locus ceruleus, solitary nucleus to the lateral funiculus to the intermediolateral cell column in the thoracic, lumbar, and sacral spine for sympathetic and parasympathetic control.

3. Flexor tracts—include the lateral reticulospinal (medullary) tract and rubrospinal tract (to upper extremities only). Extensor tracts include the medial and lateral vestibulospinal tracts and the medial (pontine) reticulospinal tract. Damage to the anterior lobe of the cerebellum removes tonic inhibition of the lateral vestibular nucleus and thus causes increased extension.

D. Spinal bones, ligaments, and joints **(Figs. A–44—A–52)**

1. Vertebrae—there are 7 cervical vertebrae (number 1 is called the **atlas** and number 2 is the **axis**), 12 thoracic vertebrae, 5 lumbar vertebrae, 5 fused sacral vertebrae, and the coccyx (may contain 3–5 fused bones).

2. Uncovertebral joints—extend between the lateral uncinate processes of the cervical vertebral bodies.

3. Anterior longitudinal ligament—extends from the basiocciput to S1 and is adherent to the vertebral bodies. The segment beween C1 and the anterior basion is called the **anterior atlanto-occipital membrane**.

4. The posterior longitudinal ligament (PLL)—extends from C1 to S1and rostrally it merges into the tectorial membrane and dura. It is thinner at the midline and is not adherent to the vertebral bodies (only to the anulus). Fat and veins lie between the PLL and the vertebral bodies. The **tectorial membrane** is the rostral extension of the PLL that is connected to the posterior basion.

5. **Transverse atlantal ligament**—extends between the tubercles of the lateral masses of the atlas and holds the dens against the anterior arch. The **superior and inferior cruciate ligaments** emerge from the transverse ligament. The superior cruciate ligament connects the transverse ligament to the posterior basion, and the inferior cruciate ligament connects the transverse ligament to the posterior body of the axis.

6. **Apical ligament**—extends from the tip of the dens to the basion.

7. **Alar ligaments**—extend from the dens to the lateral margins of the foramen magnum. There are two of them.

8. **Dentate ligaments**—extensions of pia connecting the lateral midlines of the spinal cord to the dura.

9. The normal cervical spine AP diameter at C1/2 is 15 mm and in the rest of the cervical and thoracic spine is 12 mm. The normal AP diameter in the lumbar spine is 15 to 20 mm.

10. Hemifacets for the synovial costovertebral joints are above, below, and at the tranverse processes of T1-10.

XVIII. CRANIAL FORAMINA AND MISCELLANEOUS STRUCTURES (FIGS. A-55—A-57)

A. Cribriform plate—transmits olfactory nerves and anterior and posterior ethmoidal arteries and nerves.

B. Optic canal—CN II and ophthalmic artery.

C. Superior orbital fissure—CNs III, IV, V1 (all three branches: nasociliary, frontal, and lacrimal), CN VI, sympathetic fibers from ICA plexus, superior ophthalmic vein, orbital branch of middle meningeal artery, and recurrent meningeal branch of lacrimal artery.

D. Inferior orbital fissure—CN V2, zygomatic nerve, pterygopalatine branch of maxillary nerve, infra-orbital artery and vein, and inferior ophthalmic vein.

E. Foramen rotundum—CN V2.

F. Foramen ovale—CN V3 and lesser superficial petrosal nerve.

G. Foramen spinosum—middle meningeal artery and veins.

H. Foramen lacerum—usually nothing, ICA traverses upper portion, 30% with vidian artery.

I. Carotid canal—ICA and sympathetic nerves.

J. Internal acoustic meatus—CNs VII and VIII and labyrinthine vessels.

K. Stylomastoid foramen—CN VII and stylomastoid artery.

L. Jugular foramen

    1. Pars nervosa (anteromedial) with CN IX and Jacobson's nerve.

    2. Pars venosa (posterolateral)—with internal jugular vein/jugular bulb, inferior petrosal sinus, posterior meningeal artery, CN X and XI, and Arnold's nerve.

M. Hypoglossal canal—CN XII and anterior meningeal artery.

N. Foramen magnum—spinal cord, spinal root of CN XI, vertebral arteries, and anterior and posterior spinal arteries.

O. Dorello's canal (not a true foramen)—CN VI.

P. Mandibular foramen—inferior alveolar nerve of V3.

Q. Mental foramen—mental nerve of V3 leaves mandible.

R. Incisive foramen—nasopalatine nerve (V2) and vessels to the anterior hard palate.

S. Greater palatine foramen—located medial to the third molar, transmits greater palatine nerve and vessels to the hard palate and gingiva.

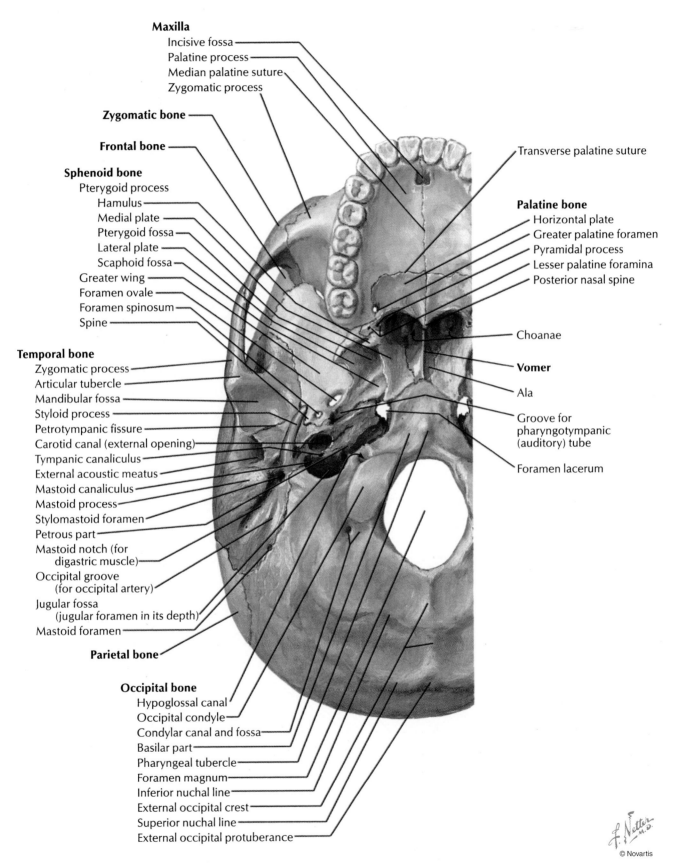

Maxilla
Incisive fossa
Palatine process
Median palatine suture
Zygomatic process

Zygomatic bone

Frontal bone

Sphenoid bone
Pterygoid process
Hamulus
Medial plate
Pterygoid fossa
Lateral plate
Scaphoid fossa
Greater wing
Foramen ovale
Foramen spinosum
Spine

Temporal bone
Zygomatic process
Articular tubercle
Mandibular fossa
Styloid process
Petrotympanic fissure
Carotid canal (external opening)
Tympanic canaliculus
External acoustic meatus
Mastoid canaliculus
Mastoid process
Stylomastoid foramen
Petrous part
Mastoid notch (for
   digastric muscle)
Occipital groove
   (for occipital artery)
Jugular fossa
   (jugular foramen in its depth)
Mastoid foramen

Parietal bone

Occipital bone
Hypoglossal canal
Occipital condyle
Condylar canal and fossa
Basilar part
Pharyngeal tubercle
Foramen magnum
Inferior nuchal line
External occipital crest
Superior nuchal line
External occipital protuberance

Transverse palatine suture

Palatine bone
Horizontal plate
Greater palatine foramen
Pyramidal process
Lesser palatine foramina
Posterior nasal spine

Choanae

Vomer

Ala

Groove for
pharyngotympanic
(auditory) tube

Foramen lacerum

© Novartis

Figure A–55   Cranial base, inferior view.

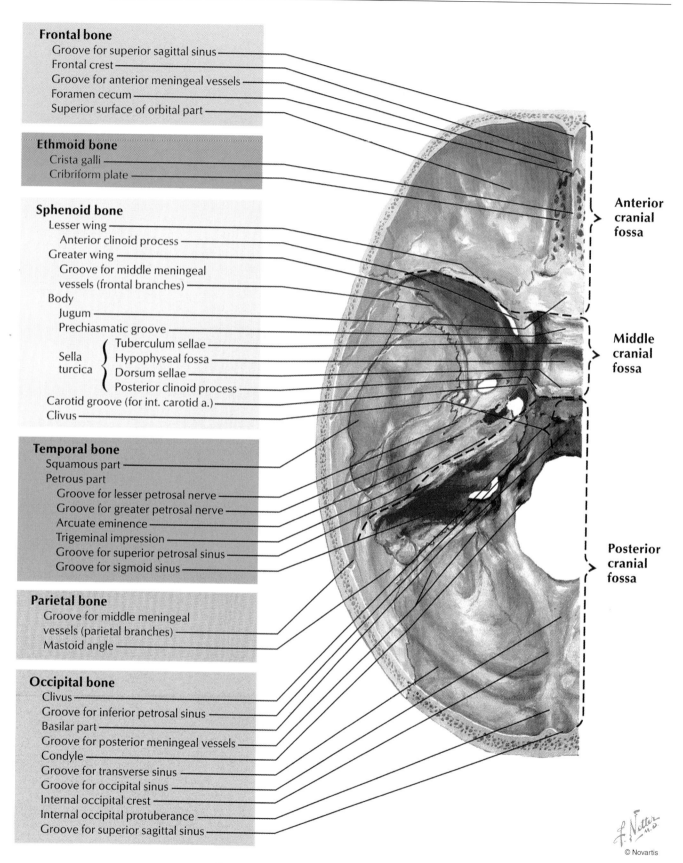

Frontal bone
Groove for superior sagittal sinus
Frontal crest
Groove for anterior meningeal vessels
Foramen cecum
Superior surface of orbital part

Ethmoid bone
Crista galli
Cribriform plate

Sphenoid bone
Lesser wing
Anterior clinoid process
Greater wing
Groove for middle meningeal
vessels (frontal branches)
Body
Jugum
Prechiasmatic groove
Sella turcica { Tuberculum sellae
Hypophyseal fossa
Dorsum sellae
Posterior clinoid process
Carotid groove (for int. carotid a.)
Clivus

Temporal bone
Squamous part
Petrous part
Groove for lesser petrosal nerve
Groove for greater petrosal nerve
Arcuate eminence
Trigeminal impression
Groove for superior petrosal sinus
Groove for sigmoid sinus

Parietal bone
Groove for middle meningeal
vessels (parietal branches)
Mastoid angle

Occipital bone
Clivus
Groove for inferior petrosal sinus
Basilar part
Groove for posterior meningeal vessels
Condyle
Groove for transverse sinus
Groove for occipital sinus
Internal occipital crest
Internal occipital protuberance
Groove for superior sagittal sinus

Anterior cranial fossa

Middle cranial fossa

Posterior cranial fossa

© Novartis

Figure A–56   Cranial base bones, superior view.

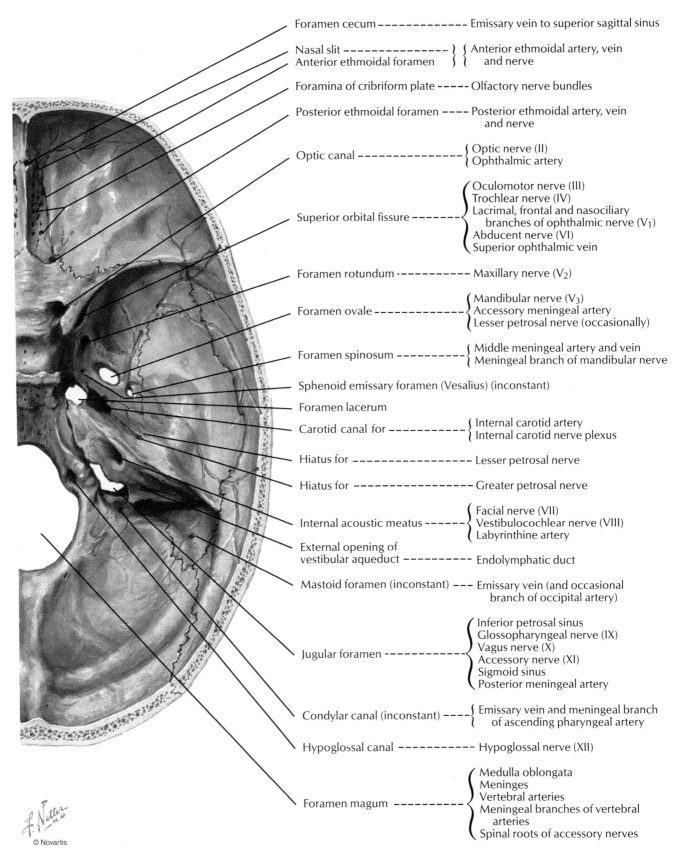

Foramen cecum –––––––––––– Emissary vein to superior sagittal sinus

Nasal slit –––––––––––––– } { Anterior ethmoidal artery, vein
Anterior ethmoidal foramen } {   and nerve

Foramina of cribriform plate ––––– Olfactory nerve bundles

Posterior ethmoidal foramen –––– Posterior ethmoidal artery, vein
                                      and nerve

Optic canal –––––––––––––– { Optic nerve (II)
                           { Ophthalmic artery

Superior orbital fissure ––––––– { Oculomotor nerve (III)
                                 { Trochlear nerve (IV)
                                 { Lacrimal, frontal and nasociliary
                                 {   branches of ophthalmic nerve (V₁)
                                 { Abducent nerve (VI)
                                 { Superior ophthalmic vein

Foramen rotundum ––––––––––– Maxillary nerve (V₂)

Foramen ovale ––––––––––– { Mandibular nerve (V₃)
                         { Accessory meningeal artery
                         { Lesser petrosal nerve (occasionally)

Foramen spinosum ––––––––– { Middle meningeal artery and vein
                          { Meningeal branch of mandibular nerve

Sphenoid emissary foramen (Vesalius) (inconstant)

Foramen lacerum

Carotid canal for ––––––––––– { Internal carotid artery
                             { Internal carotid nerve plexus

Hiatus for –––––––––––––– Lesser petrosal nerve

Hiatus for –––––––––––––– Greater petrosal nerve

Internal acoustic meatus –––––– { Facial nerve (VII)
                               { Vestibulocochlear nerve (VIII)
                               { Labyrinthine artery

External opening of
vestibular aqueduct ––––––––– Endolymphatic duct

Mastoid foramen (inconstant) ––– Emissary vein (and occasional
                                    branch of occipital artery)

Jugular foramen –––––––––– { Inferior petrosal sinus
                          { Glossopharyngeal nerve (IX)
                          { Vagus nerve (X)
                          { Accessory nerve (XI)
                          { Sigmoid sinus
                          { Posterior meningeal artery

Condylar canal (inconstant) –––– { Emissary vein and meningeal branch
                                 {   of ascending pharyngeal artery

Hypoglossal canal –––––––––– Hypoglossal nerve (XII)

Foramen magum ––––––––– { Medulla oblongata
                        { Meninges
                        { Vertebral arteries
                        { Meningeal branches of vertebral
                        {   arteries
                        { Spinal roots of accessory nerves

Figure A–57   Cranial base foramina, superior view.

T. Lesser palatine foramen—lesser palatine nerves and vessels to the soft palate.

U. Supraorbital foramen—supraorbital vessels and nerve (V1).

V. Infraorbital foramen—infraorbital vessel and nerve (V2).

W. Foramen cecum—emissary vein from superior sagittal sinus to frontal sinus and nose and anterior falcine artery. It is located between the frontal crest and crista galli.

X. Pterygopalatine fossa—contains maxillary artery, V2, pterygopalatine ganglion, and vidian nerve.

Y. Infratemporal fossa—temporalis muscle, medial and lateral pterygoid muscles, maxillary artery, pterygoid venous plexus, V3, chorda tympani nerve, otic ganglion, inferior alveolar nerve, lingual nerve, and buccal nerves.

Z. Vidian canal (pterygoid canal)—located in the base of the medial pterygoid plate of the sphenoid bone and connects the foramen lacerum to the pterygopalatine fossa, contains the vidian nerve (nerve of the pterygoid canal), which is the union of the greater superficial petrosal nerve (parasympathetic) and the deep petrosal nerve (sympathetic).

AA. Petrotympanic fissure—transmits the chorda tympani.

BB. Greater petrosal foramen—greater superficial petrosal nerve.

CC. Lesser petrosal foramen—lesser superficial petrosal nerve.

DD. Optic strut—bone between the optic foramen and superior orbital fissure.

EE. Transverse crest—bone in the internal auditory canal (porus acousticus) above the acoustic and inferior vestibular nerve (to saccule) and below the facial and superior vestibular nerve (to utricle and semicircular canals).

FF. Bill's bar—bony bar extending from the transverse crest to the roof of the porus acousticus separating the facial and superior vestibular nerves.

GG. Falciform ligament—dura extending between the anterior clinoids and the planum sphenoidale covering the optic nerves.

HH. Liliequist's membrane—two sleeves of arachnoid connecting the posteroinferior wall of the ICA cistern and the superior aspect of the interpeduncular cistern. It is attached to the medial temporal lobes laterally and the hypothalamus superiorly. It separates the basilar artery in the posterior fossa from the suprasellar cistern.

II. ICA dural rings

  1. Proximal dural ring—just distal to the exit from the cavernous sinus and is composed of a reticular layer between the oculomotor nerve and the lateral aspect of the ICA.

2. Distal dural ring—a collar of dura around the ascending vertical portion of the ICA. The ICA segment between these two rings is the "clinoidal segment" located medial to the anterior clinoid and is neither intradural nor intracavernous.

JJ. Glascock's triangle—bone overlying the petrous ICA bordered by the foramen spinosum, arcuate eminence, groove of the greater superficial petrosal nerve, and dorsal aspect of V3.

KK. Nasion—midline frontonasal suture.

LL. Glabella—most forward point on the midline supraorbital ridge.

MM. Pterion—junction of the frontal, parietal, temporal, and greater wing of sphenoid bones. It is located two fingerbreaths above the zygomatic arch and a thumb's breath behind the frontal process of the zygomatic bone.

NN. Asterion—junction of the lambdoid, occipitomastoid, and parietomastoid sutures. It lies on top of the lower $\frac{1}{2}$ of the transverse/sigmoid sinus junction.

OO. Lambda—junction of the lambdoid and sagittal sutures.

PP. Bregma—junction of coronal and sagittal sutures.

QQ. Inion—indentation under the external occipital protruberance that overlies the torcula.

RR. Opisthion—posterior margin of the foramen magnum in the midline.

SS. Sylvian fissure—locate by:

1. Marking a point $\frac{3}{4}$ of the way on a line over the superior sagittal sinus from the nasion to the inion.

2. Marking the frontozygomatic point, which is 2.5 cm up along the orbital rim above the zygomatic arch.

3. The sylvian fissure extends along the line connecting the 75% point and the frontozygomatic point. The pterion is located 3 cm behind the frontozygomatic point along the sylvian line.

TT. Rolandic fissure—locate by:

1. Upper rolandic point—2 cm posterior to the halfway point along the midline nasion/inion line.

2. Lower rolandic point—at the junction of the line from the upper rolandic point to the midzygomatic arch and the sylvian fissure line as defined previously.

3. The rolandic fissure lies between these two points. The lower rolandic point is also 2.5 cm behind the pterion along the sylvian line. The motor strip is usually 4 to 5.4 cm behind the coronal suture.

UU. Angular gyrus (part of Wernicke's area)—usually just above the pinna, although it is quite variable.

XIX. ORBIT AND TENDINOUS RING (ANULUS OF ZINN) (FIGS. A–58 AND A–59)

A. Tendinous ring—where the origins of the extraocular muscles (all but the inferior oblique) fuse to the dura/periosteum. Structures from the superior orbital fissure passing above it to the orbit include:

  1. Lacrimal nerve (V1)

  2. Frontal nerve (V1)

  3. CN IV

B. Structures from the superior orbital fissure passing through the tendinous ring to the orbit include:

  1. Superior division of CN III

  2. Nasociliary nerve (V1)

  3. Inferior division of CN III

  4. CN VI

C. Luscious (Lacrimal) French (Frontal) Tarts (Trochlear)/Stand (Superior division III) Naked (Nasociliary) In (Inferior division III) Anticipation (Adducens).

Right Orbit

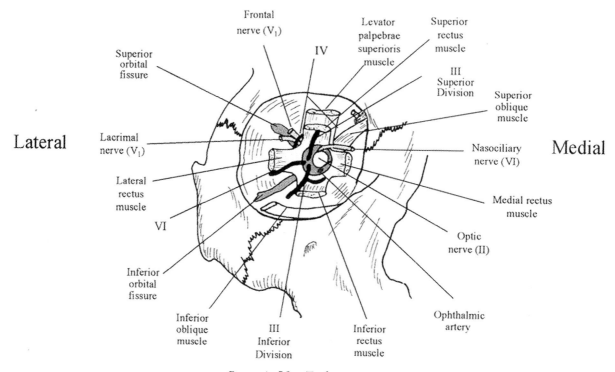

Figure A–58   Tendinous ring.

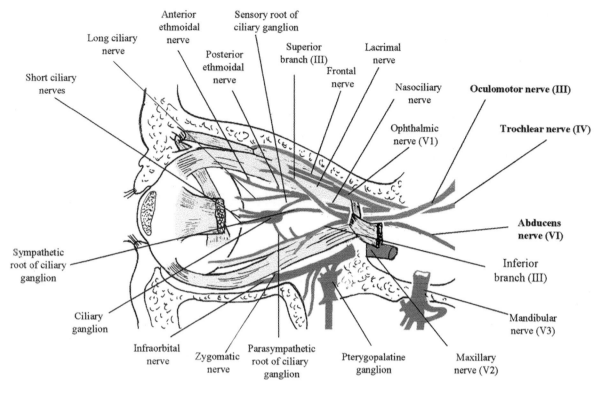

Figure A–59   Orbital schema.

D. Optic nerve and ophthalmic artery—from the optic canal and pass through the anulus of Zinn.

E. Superior and inferior ophthalmic veins—do not pass through the anulus of Zinn, but pass through the superior and inferior orbital fissures, respectively.

F. Ophthalmic artery—under CN II intracranially and the central retinal artery branches 15 mm proximal to the globe. The **central retinal artery** supplies the deeper layers of the retina. The ophthalmic artery **pial plexus** supplies CN II. The **short posterior ciliary arteries** supply the outer retinal layers, sclera, rods, and cones. The ophthalmic artery crosses over laterally to the top of CN II, and the **long posterior ciliary branches** supply the ciliary body and iris. The two dural layers split at the optic canal with one layer over the optic nerve and one layer becoming the periosteum of the orbit. The subarachnoid space extends into the globe.

XX. INNERVATION AND MUSCLES OF THE HEAD AND NECK

A. Eye—levator palpebrae superioris (superior division of CN III), superior rectus (superior division of CN III), inferior rectus (inferior division of CN III), medial rectus (inferior division of CN III), inferior oblique (inferior division of CN III), superior oblique (CN IV), lateral rectus (CN VI), and Müller's muscle (eyelid retractor, sympathetic).

B. Tympanic cavity—tensor tympani (CN V), and stapedius (CN VII).

C. Face and scalp—all innervated by CN VII.

D. Mastication—temporalis (CN V), masseter (CN V), medial pterygoid (CN V), and lateral pterygoid (CN V, only one to open mouth).

E. Tongue—all innervated by CN XII (except the palatoglossus by CN X), intrinsics and extrinsics (genioglossus, hyoglossus, and styloglossus).

F. Palate—tensor veli palatini (CN V), levator veli palatini (CN X), palatoglossus (CN X), and palatopharyngeus (CN X).

G. Pharynx—stylopharyngeus (CN IX), salpingopharyngeus (CN X), superior, middle, and inferior pharyngeal constrictors (CN X).

H. Larynx—all innervated by CN X, cricothyroid by the external branch of the superior laryngeal nerve and all others by the recurrent laryngeal nerve.

I. Neck

   1. Cervical—platysma (CN VII) and sternocleidomastoid (CN XI, C2).

   2. Suprahyoid—anterior belly of the digastric (CN V), posterior belly of the digastric (CN VII), stylohyoid (CN VII), mylohyoid (CN VII), and geniohyoid (C1 by way of CN XII).

   3. Infrahyoid—thyrohyoid (C1 by way of CN XII), sternohyoid (ansa cervicalis from C1-3), sternothyroid (ansa cervicalis), and omohyoid (ansa cervicalis).

   4. Anterior vertebral—rectus capitus anterior (C1,2), rectus capitus lateralis (C1,2), longus capitus (C1-4), and longus coli (C2-8).

   5. Lateral vertebral—anterior scalene (C5-8), middle scalene (C3,4), and posterior scalene (C3-8).

   6. Suboccipital—all from posterior rami, rectus capitus posterior major (C1), rectus capitus posterior minor (C1), obliquus capitus superior (C1), and obliquus capitus inferior (C1,2).

XXI. PERIPHERAL NERVE PLEXI

A. Cervical plexus **(Fig. A–60)**—from C1-5

   1. Sensory branches

      (a) Lesser occipital nerve (C2,3)—sensation of posterolateral scalp and around ear. The greater occipital nerve (C2) does not form a plexus because it is from the dorsal ramus.

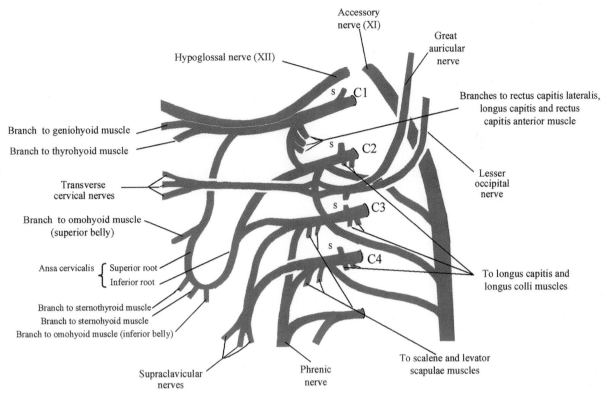

Figure A–60   Cervical plexus.

(b) Greater auricular nerve (C2,3)—sensation around ear.

(c) Transverse cutaneous nerve (C2,3)—sensation to anterior neck.

(d) Supraclavicular nerve (C3,4)—sensation to lower neck.

2. Motor branches

(a) Ansa cervicalis (C1-3, the superior root or descendens hypoglossi is from C1, and the inferior root or the descendens cervicalis is from C2,3)—Omohyoid, sternothyroid, and sternohyoid.

(b) C1 (by way of XII)—Geniohyoid and thyrohyoid.

(c) C1,2—rectus capitis lateralis, longus capitis, and rectus capitis anterior.

(d) C2-4—longus capitis and longus colli.

(e) C3,4—scalene muscles and levator scapulae.

(f) C3-5—phrenic nerve to diaphragm.

B. Brachial plexus (**Fig. A–61**)

    1. Roots (C5-T1)

        (a) C5-8—to longus colli and scalene muscles.

        (b) C5—dorsal scapular nerve to rhomboids and levator scapula.

        (c) C5-7—long thoracic nerve to serratus anterior.

    2. Trunks

        (a) Superior—suprascapular nerve to the supra and infraspinatous; nerve to subclavius muscle.

        (b) Middle—no branches.

        (c) Inferior—no branches.

    3. Divisions—no branches

    4. Cords

        (a) Lateral—lateral pectoral nerve to pectoral muscles.

        (b) Posterior—upper and lower subscapular nerves to teres major and subscapularis; thoracodorsal nerve to latissimus dorsi.

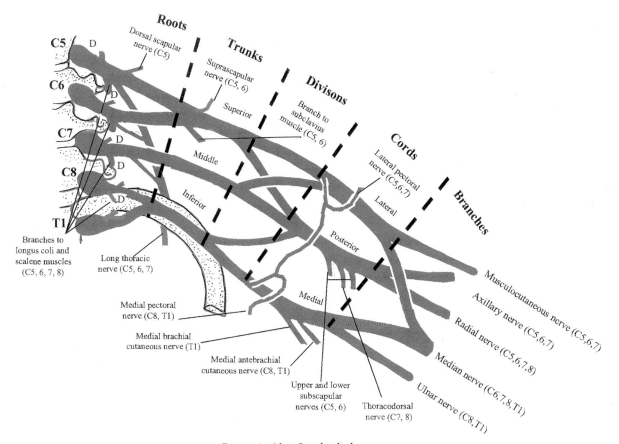

Figure A–61   Brachial plexus.

(c) Medial—medial pectoral nerve to pectoral muscles; medial brachial cutaneus nerve for the arm; medial antebrachial cutaneous nerve for the forearm.

5. Nerves

(a) Musculocutaneous—to coraco-brachialis, biceps, and brachialis.

(b) Axillary—to deltoid and teres minor.

(c) Radial—to triceps, brachioradialis, and extensor carpi radialis longus and brevis; posterior interosseus nerve to supinator, extensor carpi ulnaris, extensor digitorum, extensor digiti minimi, **abductor pollicis longus**, extensor pollicis longus and brevis, and extensor indicis.

(d) Median—pronator teres, flexor carpi radialis, palmaris longus, flexor digitorum superficialis, **abductor pollicis brevis**, **flexor pollicis brevis (also by ulnar nerve)**, opponens pollicis, and lumbricales 1 and 2. Anterior interosseus nerve to flexor digitorum profundus 1 and 2, flexor pollicis longus, and pronator quadratus.

(e) Ulnar—flexor carpi ulnaris, flexor digitorum profundus 3 and 4, abductor, opponens, and flexor digiti minimi, lumbricales 3 and 4, dorsal and palmar interosseus, **flexor pollicis brevis (also by median nerve)**, and **adductor pollicis**.

C. Lumbosacral plexus (**Fig. A–62**)—the L4 and 5 roots join medial to the psoas muscle to form the lumbosacral trunk. The S1-4 roots join in front of the pyriformis muscle and join the lumbosacral trunk to form the sacral plexus.

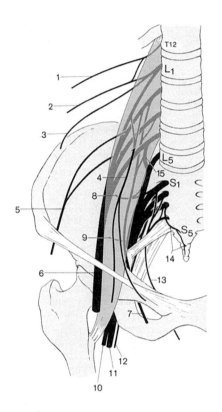

Figure A–62   Lumbosacral plexus.

1 Subcostal nerve
2–7 *Lumbar plexus*
2 Iliohypogastric nerve
3 Ilio-inguinal nerve
4 Genitofemoral nerve
5 Lateral femoral cutaneous nerve
6 Femoral nerve
7 Obturator nerve
8–13 *Sacral plexus*
8 Superior gluteal nerve
9 Inferior gluteal nerve
10, 11 Sciatic nerve
10 Peroneal portion
11 Tibial portion
12 Posterior femoral cutaneous nerve
13 Pudendal nerve
14 Coccygeal plexus
15 Lumbosacral trunk

1. Superior gluteal nerve (L4-S1)—gluteus medius and minimus and tensor fascia lata.

2. Inferior gluteal nerve (L5-S2)—gluteus maximus.

3. Femoral nerve (L2-4)—iliacus, psoas, quadraceps femoris (rectus femoris, and vastus lateralis, intermedius, and medialis), and sartorius. Also sensory from the anterior femoral cutaneous nerve to the knee and the saphenous nerve medially from the knee to the foot.

4. Obturator nerve (L2-4)—adductor brevis, adductor longus, adductor magnus (also by sciatic nerve), gracilis, and obturator externus.

5. Sciatic nerve (L4-S3, exits through the greater sciatic foramen)—semimembranosus, semitendinosus, biceps femoris, and adductor magnus (also by the obturator nerve).

    (a) Tibial nerve—to gastrocnemius, soleus, tibialis posterior, flexor hallucis longus, and flexor digitorum longus.

        (i) Medial plantar nerve—to abductor hallucis, flexor digitorum brevis, and flexor hallucis brevis.

        (ii) Lateral plantar nerve—to abductor digiti minimi, flexor digiti minimi, adductor hallucis, and interosseus muscles.

    (b) Common peroneal nerve

        (i) Superficial peroneal nerve—to peroneus longus and brevis.

        (ii) Deep peroneal nerve– to tibialis anterior, extensor digitorum longus, extensor hallucis longus, peroneus tertius, and extensor digitorum brevis.

    (c) Sensory—from the posterior femoral cutaneous nerve, the tibial nerve to most of the lower leg and the sole of the foot, and the sural nerve to a patch of the lateral foot.

6. Lateral femoral cutaneus nerve (L2,3).

7. Pudendal nerve (S2-4)—sensory to the perineum and external genitalia and motor to the external anal and urethral sphincters (from the nucleus of Onufrowicz in the anterior horn of S2-4).

8. Pelvic nerves (S2-4)—parasympathetic for bowel, bladder, and sexual function.

9. Miscellaneous sensory nerves—subcostal (T12), iliohypogastric (L1), ilioinguinal (L1), and genitofemoral (L1,2).

XXII. STRUCTURES TO MEMORIZE

A. Medial longitudinal fasciculus (MLF)—involved with eye movements with vestibular input.

B. Dorsal longitudinal fasciculus (DLF)—periventricular hypothalamus and mamillary bodies to midbrain's central gray.

C. Medial lemniscus (ML)—posterior column continuation on the way to the thalamus.

D. Lateral lemniscus—part of the auditory pathway.

E. Central tegmental tract—connects the gustatory nucleus in the rostral nucleus solitarius to the medial thalamic VPM, involved with wakefulness from the reticular formation and also carries fibers from the red nucleus to the inferior olive.

F. Medial forebrain bundle—septal area, hypothalamus, basal olfactory areas, hippocampus/subiculum to the midbrain, pons, and medulla.

G. Lamina terminalis—closed rostral end of the neural tube.

H. Stria terminalis—amygdala to hypothalamus.

I. Stria medullaris—septal area, hypothalamus, olfactory area, and anterior thalamus to habenulum.

J. Fornix—hippocampus to septal nuclei (precommissural), and hypothalamus, mamillary bodies, anterior thalamus, and cingulate gyrus (postcommissural).

K. Ansa lenticularis—GP interna to thalamus (goes around internal capsule).

L. Lenticular fasciculus (FF H2)—GP interna to thalamus (goes through internal capsule).

M. Thalamic fasciculus (FF H1)—combination of ansa lenticularis, lenticular fasciculus, and cerebellothalamic tract to the VA and VL thalamus.

N. Fasciculus retroflexus—habenulum to midbrain and interpeduncular nuclei.

O. Mamillothalamic tract—mamillary body to anterior thalamic nucleus.

P. Diagonal band of Broca—septal nuclei to amygdala.

Q. Anterior commissure—anterior part connects the two olfactory bulbs and posterior part connects the two inferior and middle frontal gyri, putamen, GP, external capsules, and claustrum.

R. Posterior commissure—crossing fibers from the pretectal nucleus for the light reflex.

S. Corpus callosum—connects most of the two hemispheres.

T. Tapetum—fibers in the corpus callosum connecting the temporal and occipital lobes.

U. Uncinate fasciculus—connects the anterior temporal lobe to the orbitofrontal gyrus.

V. Arcuate fasciculus—connects the frontal, parietal, and temporal lobes (Wernicke's area to Broca's area).

W. Medial geniculate body (MGB)—auditory relay nucleus.

X. Lateral geniculate body (LGB)—visual relay nucleus.

Y. Superior colliculus—involved with coordination of head and eye movements and the visual system.

Z. Inferior colliculus—auditory relay and processing.

AA. Superior olive—auditory relay and processing.

BB. Inferior olivary complex—cerebellar input.

CC. Ciliary ganglion—parasympathetic from oculomotor nerve.

DD. Gasserian or semilunar ganglion—trigeminal nerve.

EE. Geniculate ganglion—sensation and taste to facial nerve.

FF. Sphenopalatine ganglion (pterygopalatine)—lacrimal and nasal glands from facial nerve.

GG. Submandibular ganglion—submandibular and sublingual glands from facial nerve.

HH.   Spiral ganglion—hearing to the cochlear nerve.

II.   Scarpa's ganglion (the superior and inferior vestibular ganglia)—vestibular function to the vestibular nerve, the utricle to the superior ganglion, and the saccule to the inferior ganglion.

JJ.   Otic ganglion—parotid secretion from glossopharyngeal nerve.

KK.   Inferior ganglion of CN IX (petrosal)—taste and carotid sinus and body input to glossopharyngeal nerve.

LL.   Superior ganglion of CN IX—ear sensation to glossopharyngeal nerve.

MM.   Inferior ganglion of CN X (nodosal)—taste and visceral sensation to vagus nerve.

NN.   Superior ganglion of CN X (jugular)—ear sensation to vagus nerve.

OO.   Brachium conjunctivum—superior cerebellar peduncle.

PP.   Brachium pontis—middle cerebellar peduncle.

QQ.   Restiform and juxtarestiform bodies—inferior cerebellar peduncle.

RR.   Trapezoid body—connects the ventral cochlear nuclei to the contralateral superior olive.

SS.   Commissure of Probst—connects the nuclei of the lateral lemniscus.

TT.   Inferior collicular commissure—connects the inferior colliculi.

UU.   Short ciliary nerves—parasympathtic fibers from the ciliary ganglion to the eye, fibers enter the orbit with the inferior division of III, also contains some sympathetic fibers.

VV.   Long ciliary nerves—sympathetic fibers that emerge from the nasociliary branch of CN V1 to the eye.

WW.   Splanchnic nerves—preganglionic fibers passing through the sympathetic chain to the adrenal medulla.

XX.   Nervi erigentes—parasympathetic nerves (S2-4) to the genitals, bowel, and bladder.

YY.   Pelvic plexus and hypogastric nerves—sympathetic nerves (T10-12) to the genitals, bowel, and bladder.

ZZ.   Pudendal nerve—somatic nerve to the genitals, external anal and bladder sphincters, and perineum.

PHYSIOLOGY

I. CELLULAR MOLECULAR TRANSPORT

A. Cell membrane—a lipid bilayer that contains channel and carrier proteins to regulate the flow of ions and other molecules.

B. Simple diffusion—occurs either directly through the lipid bilayer of the membrane or through protein channels. Some molecules are very lipid soluble (i.e., O_2, N_2, CO_2, and ETOH). Small molecules like H_2O can bullet directly through the membrane. Ions pass poorly because (1) they attract many H_2O molecules and become larger hydrated ions and (2) they bounce off the positive and negative charges in the lipid bilayer. Glucose passes poorly because it is too large. Simple diffusion also occurs through protein channels that are highly selective for specific ions or molecules because of the channel shape and charge.

C. Selective permeability—limits which ions may diffuse through certain channels. Na^+ channels are small and have a negative charge inside. Once the ion is inside the channel, it can diffuse out in either direction. K^+ channels have no negative charge and no force pulling K^+ ions away from H_2O molecules hydrating them, but they are smaller than hydrated Na^+ molecules. The small size of the ion pore may create selectivity.

D. Gating of a channel—when a protein shape change opens or closes the passage for ion transport.

E. Voltage-gated channels—where the conformation of the gate and thus ion passage depends on the electrical potential of the cell membrane. If it is highly negative inside the cell, the Na^+ gate is closed. When the membrane becomes less negative, the gate opens. The K^+ gate opens when the inside of the cell is positively charged. An individual channel has an "all-or-none" response so it is either completely open or closed.

F. Ligand-gated channels—open with the binding of a certain molecule to the receptor protein, such as when acetylcholine (ACh) binds the ACh receptor.

G. Facilitated diffusion—carrier-mediated transport. A molecule binds a receptor protein, which undergoes a configuration change that carries it inside the cell and releases it, and then the receptor protein reverts to its original shape. The rate of diffusion depends on the number of receptors and the rate of the configuration change. It is maximal when all carrier proteins are filled. Molecules may diffuse in either direction. Facilitated diffusion is used for the transport of glucose and various amino acids.

H. Net rate of diffusion—occurs in a direction influenced by the molecular permeability, the concentration gradient, and the electrical potential difference (only with ions). A steady state is reached when the electrical forces and the concentration forces balance. The electrochemical gradient is the sum of the electrical, concentration, and pressure forces. No molecule can diffuse against it.

I. Active transport—uses energy to move molecules such as Na^+, K^+, Ca^{++}, Fe^{++}, H^+, Cl^-, I^-, uric acid, sugars, and most amino acids across membranes.

J. Primary active transport—uses ATP-derived energy for the transport of Na^+, K^+, Ca^{++}, H^+, and Cl^-. The **Na^+/K^+ pump** has a carrier segment with two proteins. The larger protein has three receptor sites on the intracellular side for Na^+, and the smaller one has two receptor sites on the extracellular side for K^+. The intracellular part has ATPase activity. **One ATP moves three Na^+ ions out of the cell and two K^+ ions in.** This electrogenic pump creates a charge difference across the membrane.

K. Secondary active transport—uses an existing ionic gradient created by previous ATP cleavage to transport a molecule against an electrochemical gradient. It requires a carrier protein.

L. Cotransport—where a Na^+ ion (or other ion) enters the cell and pulls another molecule in with it down the electrochemical gradient. The membrane carrier protein only makes the needed configuration change when both molecules bind.

M. Countertransport—where a Na^+ ion (or other ion) binds the carrier protein from outside the cell and an intracellular ion or molecule binds it on the inside. As the Na^+ ion enters the cell, the other ion or molecule is removed.

II. MEMBRANE POTENTIALS AND ACTION POTENTIALS

A. Membrane potential—created by selective permeability to Na^+ and K^+ ions.

B. Nernst potential (for 1 ion) $= \pm 61 \log C_i/C_o$. C_i is the intracellular ion concentration and C_o is the extracellular ion concentration. The $\pm$ is positive when the ion is negative and negative when the ion is positive (Table P–1).

TABLE P–1. MEMBRANE POTENTIAL

Ion	Extracellular (mEq/L)	Intracellular (mEq/L)	Eq potential (mV)
Na^+	142	14	+61
K^+	4	140	−94
Cl^-	103	4	−86
Ca^{++}	2.4	0.0001	+267

C. **Equilibrium potential** of an ion—the membrane potential at which no net diffusion occurs because of balanced electrical and chemical gradients. The potential outside the membrane is always 0 by definition.

D. Goldman equation—used to determine the potential for many ions: $EMV = -61 \log(Na^+$ concentrationinside $\times$ permeability $+ [K^+]i \times Perm + [Cl^-]i \times Perm)/(Na$ concentration outside $\times$ permeability $+ [K^+]o \times Perm + [Cl^-]o \times Perm)$. It is proportional to electrical charge, concentration, and permeability. The membrane functions as a capacitor to store charge.

E. **Resting membrane potential (RMP)** $= -90\,\text{mV}$ in large myelinated peripheral nerves and in skeletal muscle. It is determined mainly by the potential of K^+ ($-94\,\text{mV}$) because K^+ is 100 times more permeable than Na^+. The Na^+ potential is $+61\,\text{mV}$. Ca^{++} ions are not very permeable, so they have little effect on the RMP. The final potential is the sum of the $-86\,\text{mV}$ by diffusion through Na^+ and K^+ leak channels and the $-4\,\text{mV}$ by the Na^+/K^+ ATP pump. The RMP of a large peripheral nerve fiber or a skeletal muscle fiber is $-90\,\text{mV}$; of the soma of a neuron it is $-65\,\text{mV}$; and of small nerve fibers and smooth muscle it is $-55\,\text{mV}$.

F. Action potential—when a rapid change in the membrane potential alters conductance through Na^+ and K^+ voltage-gated channels. The resting membrane potential starts at $-90\,\text{mV}$. First, **Na^+ permeability increases** causing the membrane to depolarize to $+35\,\text{mV}$ in large fibers and $0\,\text{mV}$ in smaller fibers. It repolarizes in 1/10,000th of a second as the Na^+ channels close and the **K^+ channels open**.

G. Positive after-potential—the overshoot repolarization to $-100\,\text{mV}$.

H. Na^+ and K^+ permeability changes with the action potential, although **Cl^- permeability does not change much**.

I. Only a small number of ions present in the cell need to cross the membrane (1/100,000,000) to cause the -90 to $+35\,\text{mV}$ change.

J. At rest, **K^+ conductance is higher** than Na^+ conductance because the membrane leaks the K^+ ions more than the Na^+ ions.

K. Initiation of an action potential—requires a sudden rise of 15 to 30 mV to reach a **$-65\,\text{mV}$ threshold**.

L. The action potential in the neuron starts at the **axon hillock** because there are seven times more voltage-gated Na^+ channels there, so it is more easily depolarized than the soma. A $+30\,\text{mV}$ rise is required at the soma, whereas only a $+20\,\text{mV}$ rise is needed at the hillock to decrease the membrane potential to $-45\,\text{mV}$. The potential is evenly distributed in the soma.

M. The action potential requires approximately 40 to 80 excitatory post-synaptic potentials (EPSPs). Inhibitory post-synaptic potentials (IPSPs) open **K^+ or Cl^- channels**, while ESPSs open Na^+ channels.

N. The Nernst equation value for Cl^- is $-86\,\text{mV}$, whereas the soma's potential is $-65\,\text{mV}$, so Cl^- will move inside to increase the negativity and hyperpolarize the membrane.

O. Accommodation of a membrane to a stimulus occurs by a slow rise in the membrane potential that allows some Na^+ gates to deactivate while others open. This causes the membrane to need either a larger depolarization or a faster rise of depolarization to trigger an action potential.

P. Propagation of an action potential—occurs because the adjacent segment has a potential change. The ion channels open and the impulse moves ahead in both directions. The velocity of the action potential increases with **increased transmembrane resistance**, **decreased internal resistance**, and **decreased membrane capacitance**. Myelin increases transmembrane resistance and decreases membrane capacitance.

Q. Voltage-gated Na^+ channels—have an activation gate on the outside and an inactivation on the inside. At resting membrane potential, the inactivation gate is open and activation gate is closed. The activation gate opens at -70 to -50 mV and allows Na^+ to pour in. Both gates open for a few 10,000ths of a second, then the inactivation gates close more slowly than the activation gates open. The inactivation gate does not open again until the membrane potential returns to the resting state and the activation gates are closed.

R. Voltage-gated K^+ channels—open slowly as the membrane depolarizes so that K^+ efflux occurs as the Na^+ inactivation gate closes.

S. **Tetrodotoxin**—blocks Na^+ channels. **TEA** blocks voltage-gated K^+ channels.

T. Cl^- ions—passively leak in, but **little change in flow occurs with the action potential**. The concentration of Cl^- ions is low inside because the -90 mV resting membrane potential charge repels them. The Nernst equation value is -86 mV so it is not actively pumped.

U. Ca^{++} (and $Ca^{++} + Na^+$) channels—slow channels, unlike the fast Na^+ channels. When less Ca^{++} is in the interstitial fluid, Na^+ channels open sooner (-80 mV) so the membrane is more excitable and may reach **tetany**. Possibly, Ca^{++} ions bind to the Na^+ channel protein and force it to require higher voltage to open.

V. During the action potential, many negatively charged molecules remain intracellular (i.e., proteins, phosphates, sulfates).

W. Patch clamps—record ion current flow across membranes. They have micropipettes with diameters of 1 to 2 μm, with a membrane patch either on or off of the cell. One can "clamp" the system to set a voltage. Patch clamps can record multiple or single channels.

X. Heart muscle—has a longer depolarization with a plateau phase because of the fast voltage-gated Na^+ channels, **slow voltage-gated Ca^{++} channels** (mainly Ca^{++}, but some Na^+), and also the K^+ channels that do not open until the end of the plateau.

Y. Rhythmicity—repetitive self-induced discharges of cardiac muscle, smooth muscle, and some neurons. It occurs because of a decreased threshold for action potential. The membrane must be permeable to Na^+ ions even in a resting state. The resting membrane potential is -60 to -70 mV and some Na^+ and Ca^{++} gates remain open at rest. The delay in subsequent depolarization is due to an overshoot of K^+ efflux causing hyperpolarization. As the K^+ conductance decreases, the membrane depolarizes, and then the K^+ conductance increases. The action potential occurs when the K^+ conductance is at its lowest.

Z. Myelin—contains sphingomyelin. Peripheral nerves have twice as many unmyelinated as myelinated fibers. **Nodes of Ranvier** are unmyelinated segments that occur every 1 to 3 mm and are 3 μm long. **Saltatory conduction** occurs between nodes. It is faster, uses less energy, and has faster repolarization (less ions to move) than nonsaltatory conduction. Repolarization is so fast that K^+ channels do not contribute much, so it is **mainly by Na^+ channels closing**.

AA.   Conduction velocity—in small unmyelinated nerves. It is around 0.5 m/s and in large myelinated nerves is up to **120 m/s**.

BB.   Excitation of a cell—occurs by either a mechanical disturbance to a membrane (i.e., pressure or stretch of the skin), a chemical interaction (interneurons and some sensory receptors), or an electrical interaction (in excitable cells such as neurons or cardiac or smooth muscle cells, and many others).

CC.   **Refractory period**—when Na^+ channels (and some Ca^{++} channels) are not reversed and remain closed until the membrane repolarizes and some K^+ channels still remain open, causing hyperpolarization. During the **absolute refractory period**, the neuron will not fire. It lasts 1/2500th of a second in large myelinated fibers. During the **relative refractory period**, the neuron needs a supranormal stimulus to fire. It lasts $\frac{1}{4}$ to $\frac{1}{2}$ as long as the absolute refractory period.

DD.   **Membrane stabilizers**—decrease excitability. They include increased serum Ca^{++}, decreased serum K^+ (familial periodic paralysis), local anesthetics (i.e., procaine), acidosis (pH $<$ 7.0), and hypoxia. **Membrane destabilizers** increase excitability. They include decreased serum Ca^{++}, increased serum K^+, alkalosis (pH $>$ 7.8, and therefore seizures are induced by hyperventilation), caffeine, and strychnine.

III. SYNAPSES AND NEUROTRANSMITTERS

A.   Synapses—either transmit an impulse, block an impulse, change an impulse from single to repetitive, or integrate it with other impulses.

B.   Chemical synapses—the most frequent type in the CNS. They have unidirectional flow. About 40 neurotransmitters have been identified.

C.   Electrical synapses—use direct current spread from one cell to another by tubular protein channels forming gap junctions between cells allowing ions to pass through. They are found in cardiac and smooth muscle but are rare in the mammalian CNS. They have bidirectional flow.

D.   Eighty to ninety-five percent of axons synapse with dendrites and 5 to 20% with the soma.

E.   Synaptic cleft—20 to 30 nm wide.

F.   Presynaptic terminals—contain synaptic vesicles and mitochondria to make ATP for neurotransmitter synthesis. The membrane has many voltage-gated Ca^{++} channels that open with depolarization, and the influx of Ca^{++} ions causes neurotransmitter release. Possibly, the Ca^{++} ions bind release sites inside the terminal membrane and vesicles bind there and fuse. Exocytosis involves the release of a few vesicles per action potential. Each vesicle contains **10,000 molecules of acetylcholine (ACh) or 1 quantum**. The release of 1 quantum causes **a miniature end-plate potential (MEPP)**. After the action potential, Ca^{++} ions are removed from the presynaptic terminal by active transport, bound to cytosol proteins, and transported to storage vesicles. After fusing with the membrane, vesicles reform on the inside.

G. Presynaptic inhibition—occurs by decreased flow of Ca^{++} into the presynaptic terminal by either blocking Ca^{++} channels or inhibiting voltage-gated Na^+ channels. This mechanism of inhibition is slower but longer lasting than postsynaptic inhibition.

H. Postsynaptic neurons—have receptors with a binding component and an ionophore component. Either a chemically activated ion channel or an enzyme activates an internal reaction. Chemically activated ion channels include Na^+ (opening causes excitement), K^+ and Cl^- (opening causes inhibition).

I. Enzyme receptors—may use cAMP, may activate cellular genes or protein kinases, may increase or decrease the number of receptors, and may alter the reactivity of the synapses. Neurotransmitters that do this are modulators and may be used for various functions such as memory.

J. **Excitation**—occurs by opening Na^+ channels, closing K^+ or Cl^- channels, altering receptors to increase excitation or decrease inhibition, and changing intracellular activity.

K. **Inhibition**—occurs by opening K^+ or Cl^- channels or changing receptors.

L. Summation—the additive effect of EPSPs and IPSPs. They cause increased or decreased ion permeability that lasts for 1 to 2 ms and returns to baseline in 15 ms. Each axon terminal releases substances that cause a 0.5 to 1 mV change, but 20 mV is needed to reach the depolarization threshold necessary to fire an action potential. **Spatial summation** occurs when different parts of the neuron are stimulated simultaneously. **Temporal summation** is the additive effect of postsynaptic potentials over time. A neuron is considered "facilitated" if an EPSP puts it closer to threshold. Many dendrites are unable to generate action potentials because they have too few voltage-gated channels, but the current can spread to the axon by means of the cytosol. Decremented conduction occurs because the membrane potential changes more distal on the dendrite have less effect on the soma because current leaks out along the way. Dendrites do not get the spread of an action potential like the axon and soma so they may start to accumulate EPSPs sooner.

M. Fatigue—when repetitive stimulation causes a decreased frequency of discharges. This is protective against excessive neuronal activity. It occurs (1) by exhaustion of neurotransmitter stores in the presynaptic terminals (only 10,000 transmissions are loaded at once), (2) by progressive inactivation of postsynaptic receptors, and (3) by the buildup of postsynaptic Ca^{++} that opens Ca^{++} activated K^+ channels to hyperpolarize the membrane.

N. Posttetanic facilitation—occurs after repetitive impulses followed by rest. Synapses become more responsive because of increased Ca^{++} in the presynaptic terminals (slowly pumped out), causing increased neurotransmitter release. This has been postulated to be the mechanism of short-term memory.

O. Synaptic delay—the minimum time from presynaptic to postsynaptic terminals in an action potential and usually equals 0.5 ms.

P. Different neurons have different thresholds for excitation, baseline RMPs, and different frequency of discharges.

Q. Approximately 40 neurotransmitters are known. Only one small molecule type of neurotransmitter is released per neuron, but a neuron may also release more than one neuropeptide.

R. **Small molecule neurotransmitters**—rapid acting and account for most of the acute reactions in the CNS. They are made in the cytosol of presynaptic terminals and actively transported into vesicles. A few vesicles are released per action potential. They usually act at ion channels. They are inactivated in milliseconds by diffusion, enzymatic destruction, and active transport into presynaptic terminals (re-uptake).

1. Three classes of small molecule neurotransmitters—class 1 is acetylcholine (ACh). Class 2 are amines (i.e., norepinephrine [NE], epinephrine [EPI], dopamine [DA], serotonin, and histamine). Class 3 are amino acids (i.e., GABA, glycine, glutamate, and aspartate).

   (a) ACh—usually excitatory, made in the nerve terminal from acetyl-CoA and choline, split at the synapse by acetylcholinesterase, and the choline is reabsorbed. It is found in the motor cortex, skeletal muscle, preganglionic autonomic nerves, postganglionic parasympathetic nerves, and postganglionic sympathetic nerves to sweat glands.

   (b) NE—usually excitatory and found in the pontine locus ceruleus and postganglionic sympathetic nerves.

   (c) DA—inhibitory and found in the neurons in the substantia nigra (SN) that project to the putamen and caudate nuclei. Synthesis is from tyrosine to DOPA (uses tyrosine hydroxylase, the rate-limiting step) to DA to NE to EPI.

   (d) Glycine—inhibitory and found in the spinal cord (especially in Renshaw cells).

   (e) GABA—inhibitory and found in the cortex, basal ganglia, cerebellum (Purkinje's cells), and spinal cord.

   (f) Glutamate—excitatory and found in the cortex, dentate gyrus of the hippocampus, striatum, and cerebellar granule cells.

   (g) Serotonin—inhibitory and found in the median raphe nucleus. It is involved with decreasing pain, increasing sleep, and altering mood. It is used by the pineal gland to synthesize melatonin that is released in a diurnal rhythm.

2. Small molecule neurotransmitter receptors

   (a) Acetylcholine receptors

      (i) **Nicotinic receptors**—stimulated by nicotine. They are located in the neuromuscular junction (NMJ) and preganglionic endings of both sympathetic and parasympathetic fibers. The automonic nicotinic receptors have five subunits $\alpha_2\beta\gamma\delta$. The α-subunit is the binding site for ACh (thus each receptor can bind two ACh molecules) and is composed of four hydrophobic transmembrane proteins. Stimulation of the receptor elicits a fast EPSP. The receptor is blocked by hexamethonium (depolarizing, not reversible with anticholinesterase). The nicotinic receptor at the NMJ has only two subunits, and stimulation of the receptor elicits a slow EPSP (opens Na^+ and Ca^{++} channels) and a slow IPSP (opens K^+ channels).

      (ii) **Muscarinic receptors**—stimulated by Muscarine. They are located in all of the postganglionic parasympathetic endings and the postganglionic sympathetic endings to **sweat glands**. The receiver's effect is mediated by a **G protein** with a secondary messenger system. Activation of one G protein will inhibit all other G proteins in the cell. This receptor is blocked by pertussis toxin.

(b) Adrenergic receptors—norepinephrine stimulates alpha $>$ beta. Epinephrine stimulates alpha and beta equally. See Chapter 6 for more detail.

(c) GABA receptor—increases **Cl^-** channel permeability. The GABA receptor has five subunits, with a central Cl^- channel ($\alpha_2 \beta_2$ and γ or δ). The type A receptor is more common and causes a rapid increase in Cl^- conductance. The type B receptor uses a G protein as a secondary messenger. The GABA-A receptor's α-subunit binds benzodiazepines and GABA, whereas the β-subunit binds GABA. Both barbiturates and benzodiazepines are type A agonists, whereas baclofen is a type B agonist. The GABA receptor is blocked by picrotoxin (causes seizures).

(d) Glutmate receptors—most linked with **cell death** (by Ca^{++} influx) and synaptic plasticity. There are ligand-gated only (metabotropic) and both ligand and voltage-gated (NMDA, AMPA, kainate) types. Some are blocked by Mg^{++}. The **NMDA receptor** is one type of glutamate receptor. It is voltage regulated because at normal RMP, Mg^{++} blocks the channel, whereas with depolarization, the Mg^{++} is driven out and the channel opens. It is also ligand-gated by glutamate, permeable to Ca^{++}, and requires glycine as a coagonist for activation. Non-NMDA receptors do not need glycine for activation. The NMDA, kainate, and AMPA/quisqualate receptors are all permeable to monovalent cations (Na^+ and K^+).

(e) Glycine receptor—involves **Cl^-** channels and binds strychnine (blocks **Renshaw** activity and increases muscle rigidity).

(f) GABA and glycine receptors—permeable to Cl^-.

(g) DA receptor—the D1 receptor uses cAMP.

S. **Neuropeptide neurotransmitters**—large and slow acting, made in the soma, and packaged by the endoplasmic reticulum and Golgi apparatus after being split into smaller parts. They are transported to the tips of the axon by means of axonal streaming at a rate of a few centimeters per day. The vesicles are not recycled. Less are released, but they are much more potent and have a longer action then small molecule neurotransmitters. They close Ca^{++} channels and change metabolic machinery and receptors. They diffuse into tissues and are destroyed within minutes to hours. They include hypothalamic-releasing hormones, pituitary peptides, CCK, and bradykinin.

T. Intracellular second messengers

1. cAMP—increased with D1 receptor stimulation.

2. cGMP—involved with photoreception and is increased by nitric oxide.

3. IP_3—hydrolyzed by phospholipase C and opens the Ca^{++} channels in the ER to increase Ca^{++} influx into the cytosol.

4. DAG—synergistically activates protein kinase C with Ca^{++}.

5. Ca^{++}—binds calmodulin.

6. G proteins—see Section VII.

U. Axonal transport—can be slow (a few millimeters per day) or fast (200 to 400 mm/d, using microtubules) and anterograde or retrograde (only slow type). Dynein is the motor protein for retrograde fast transport. Dynamin uses GTP for energy.

IV. SENSORY RECEPTORS

A. Sensory receptors

1. Mechanoreceptors—sense deformation.

2. Thermoreceptors—sense temperature change with some specific for heat and others for cold.

3. Nociceptors—create pain in the presence of tissue damage or physical or chemical changes.

4. Electromagnetic receptors—detect the light in the retina.

5. Chemoreceptors—detect various chemicals for taste, smell, arterial oxygen and carbon dioxide, blood osmolarity, and so forth.

B. Labeled-line principle —different sensory modalities terminate in different parts of the brain.

C. When the receptor potential rises above threshold, an action potential is generated. A higher receptor potential elicits increased action potential frequency but no change in amplitude. The receptor potential is **graded and nonpropagated**, whereas the action potential is a propagated all-or-none response.

D. Receptor membranes develop potential changes by different mechanisms:

1. Mechanoreceptors—react as deformation stretches the membrane and opens ion channels.

2. Chemical receptors—stimulated by certain chemicals that open ion channels.

3. Temperature receptors—react to temperature changes by opening ion channels directly or changing the membrane ion permeability.

4. Electromagnetic energy—may open ion channels directly or change membrane ion permeability.

EXAMPLE: A pacinian corpuscle is composed of a central nerve fiber with surrounding capsule layers. Compression causes changes in the central fiber by elongation, bending, denting, and so forth. As the unmyelinated tip of the fiber deforms, the Na^+ conductance increases, a receptor potential is generated, and an action potential is produced if the receptor potential is large enough. The frequency of the action potential is proportional to the amplitude of the receptor potential and plateaus at high levels.

E. Adaptation—when continuous sensory stimulation causes the receptor to decrease its firing rate.

EXAMPLE: A pacinian corpuscle adapts by:

1. After the initial pressure wave, the fluid is evenly distributed so the firing ceases even though the corpuscle is still compressed and another signal forms when the compression is removed. Adaptation occurs here in $1/100$ s.

2. Accommodation by the gradual inactivation of Na^+ channels; this adaptation is much slower. Both the receptor and terminal nerve fibers adapt.

F. Pacinian corpuscles and hair receptors are phasic receptors. They increase their firing rate with an increased rate of change and adapt rapidly.

G. Joint capsules, muscle spindles, vestibular maculae, pain receptors, baroreceptors, chemoreceptors, Ruffini's end organs, and Merkel's discs are tonic receptors. They adapt slowly, transmit impulses for many hours, and may rarely adapt to extinction.

H. Mechanoreceptors may adapt completely. Pain receptors tend to adapt less and chemoreceptors are variable.

V. NERVE TRANSMISSION

A. Nerve fibers or axons are 0.2 to 20 μm in diameter. The velocity of transmission ranges from 0.5 to 120 m/s, with the larger fibers conducting faster. The largest fibers can conduct an impulse the length of a football field in a second, and the thinnest may require 2 seconds to conduct from the big toe to the spinal cord.

B. Nerve fiber types

1. **IA** (Aα)—muscle spindle (primary or annulospiral ending), largest and fastest (120 m/s) fibers.

2. **IB** (Aα)—muscle tendon (Golgi tendon organ).

3. **II** (Aβ and Aγ)—muscle spindle (secondary or flower-spray ending) and cutaneous tactile receptors.

4. III (**A$_\delta$**)—temperature, crude touch, and pricking pain.

5. IV (**C**)—unmyelinated fibers carrying pain, itch, temperature, and crude touch.

C. Motor fibers

1. Skeletal muscle—**A$_\alpha$** (fastest).

2. Muscle spindle—**A$_\gamma$** .

3. Sympathetic—**C** (unmyelinated, slowest).

D. Receptive field of a nerve fiber—the surface area it innervates. Each nerve fiber has multiple endings, and most are in the center of the field. Each stimulus may hit more than one fiber.

E. Spatial summation of a stimulus—the more intense stimulus hits more nerve endings and stimulates more fibers.

F. Temporal summation—as an increased stimulus intensity causes an increased rate of neuronal firing.

G. A neuronal pool—the neurons in a pathway that have a certain stimulatory field. They connect with many other neurons, but most are in the center of the field. The input fiber may have enough branches to be suprathreshold in the center of the field and subthreshold but facilitated on the periphery. The central zone that is stimulated or inhibited by a fiber is the liminal or stimulated zone, and the peripheral zone is the subthreshold or subliminal zone.

H. Divergence—where an incoming fiber hits many other cells and may amplify a signal in one tract (i.e., one motor neuron stimulating 10,000 muscle fibers) or multiple tracts (i.e., dorsal column input into the cerebellum and cortex).

I. Convergence—where many different fibers give input to one neuron, either from similar or different sources. Rarely one neuron creates enough stimulation of a single postsynaptic neuron to elicit an action potential (i.e., Purkinje's cells to the deep nuclei in the cerebellum).

J. Reciprocal inhibitory circuit—where an axon branch stimulates an interneuron to inhibit an antagonist muscle while stimulating an agonist muscle.

K. Afterdischarge—where lingering stimulus input (especially with long-acting neurotransmitters) may elicit repetitive action potentials after the initial signal has gone.

L. Oscillatory circuit (reverberatory)—where the output of the circuit feeds back and restimulates itself. A longer cycle occurs if more interneurons are used. They stop by fatigue of a synapse. Continuous signal output occurs by (1) neuronal excitability caused by low RMP (cerebellum and spinal cord interneurons) and (2) reverberating circuits in which input may cause an increase or decrease in the action potential frequency (autonomic). Rhythmic signal output is by reverberating circuits, such as the respiratory center of the pons and medulla.

M. Stabilization of nervous function is needed because if all the connections proceeded forward, a seizure would be induced. The nervous system inhibits excessive spread by (1) feedback circuits onto itself or other inhibitory pools and (2) fatigue of synapses by ion changes (short term) and upgrading or downgrading of receptor proteins (long term).

VI. SOMATIC SENSATIONS

A. Tactile sensations—touch, pressure, vibration, and tickle. Touch, pressure, and vibration use the same receptors.

B. Somatic sensory receptors

   1. **Free nerve endings**—pain, touch, and pressure.

   2. **Meissner's corpuscles**—touch. These are rapidly adapting, located in the dermal papillae of the nonhairy skin of fingertips and lips, have small fields, and are carried by large Aβ myelinated fibers.

3. **Merkel's discs** (expanded tip tactile receptors)—touch and pressure. They are slowly adapting, have small receptive fields, and are located in the dermal papillae of hairy and nonhairy skin. Many Merkel's discs fill one Iggo dome receptor under the epithelium that is innervated by a single Aβ myelinated fiber.

4. **Pacinian corpuscles** —vibration (high-frequency stimulation). These are rapidly adapting and are located in the superficial and deep tissue.

5. **Ruffini end organs**—heavy touch and pressure. These are slowly adapting, located in the deep layers (subcutaneous tissue and joint capsules), and have large receptive fields.

6. Hair end organ for touch—these are rapidly adapting and located at the base of a hair follicle.

7. Superficial location—Meissner's corpuscles (touch) and Merkel's discs (pressure).

8. Deep location—Pacinian corpuscles (touch and pressure).

9. Slowly adapting—Merkel's discs and Ruffini's end organs.

10. Rapidly adapting—Meissner's corpuscles and pacinian corpuscles.

C. Somatic nerve fibers

1. Touch sensation—mostly carried by Aβ fibers at speeds of 30 to 70 m/s. Free nerve endings transmit some touch by means of Aδ myelinated fibers at speeds of 5 to 30 m/s and C unmyelinated fibers at speeds of < 2 m/s (tickle). Crude pressure, poorly localized touch, and tickle are carried by smaller, slower fibers occupying less space in the nerve bundle.

2. Vibration—carried by Aβ fibers. All tactile receptors are involved but each at different frequencies: Pacinian corpuscles at 30 to 800 cycles/s and Meissner's corpuscles at 80 cycles/s.

3. Tickle and itch—use free nerve endings located in the superficial skin and carried by C fibers. Itch impulses decrease if the stimulant is removed (a fly) or with scratching that causes pain, which causes produces inhibition.

4. Pain—uses free nerve endings and is carried by C fibers. See the following sections for more detail.

5. Peripheral sensory or mixed nerves—contain four times more unmyelinated than myelinated fibers. The unmyelinated fibers are C fibers and autonomic postganglionic efferents. The myelinated fibers are Aδ, touch, and pressure. Proprioceptive fibers travel with motor nerves. Each axon connects to several receptors of one type.

D. **Anterolateral** ascending sensory system—contains smaller myelinated fibers that conduct at speeds of 2 to 40 m/s. It senses warm, cold, pain, crude touch, tickle, itch, and sexual stimulation. These sensations do not require discrete localization, so they have poor spatial localization, poor intensity grading, and poor rapid signal repetition. Crude touch originates from the receptors to the DRG (primary cells) to the spinal cord in laminae 1, 4, 5, and 6 in the dorsal horns. Fibers ascend in the anterior (ipsilateral) and lateral (contralateral by crossing in the **anterior commissure** within three levels) spinothalamic tracts to the **VPL (body), VPM (face)**, and posterior thalamic nuclei for touch and temperature sensation. Fibers also travel in the spinoreticular tract to the **intralaminar thalamic nucleus** for pain.

E. **Dorsal column** system—contains large myelinated fibers that conduct at speeds of 30 to 110 m/s. It senses fine touch, vibration, position, and pressure. It has more spatial orientation of fibers (somatotopic organization).

  1. Axons from the DRG (with the primary nerve cell bodies) enter the spinal cord and divide into a medial branch that travels up the dorsal column (25% of fibers) and a lateral branch (75% of fibers) with multiple synapses in the dorsal horn for reflexes. The second-order neurons are in the medulla at the **nuclei gracilis** (lower limbs, medial) and **cuneatus** (upper limbs, lateral). The arcuate fibers cross to form the **medial lemniscus (ML)** and join fibers from the main sensory nucleus of V and the upper spinal nucleus of V to end in the thalamic VPL (body) and VPM (face).

  2. The ventrobasal complex (VPL, VPM, and the posterior thalamic nucleus) sends fibers to the cortical somatosensory areas SS1 and SS2. A somatotopic organization exists with the **lower limbs medial in the spinal cord, lateral in the thalamus, and medial again in the cortex**.

  3. Position sense—static proprioception and kinesthetic proprioception to detect joint angles in all directions and the rate of change.

  4. Proprioceptive impulses—start at the muscle spindles, the Pacinian corpuscles, Ruffini's end organs, and Golgi tendon organs of the extremities. Lower limb proprioception is carried in the **lateral column** from the **Clarke's column** neurons through the **dorsal spinocerebellar** tract to the cerebellum, **not in the posterior columns**. Upper extremity proprioception travels through the posterior columns in the fasciculus cuneatus before synapsing in the **accessory cuneate nucleus** in the caudal medulla before going to the cerebellum.

F. The sensory cortex—arranged in vertical columns, with a diameter of 0.4 mm, containing 10,000 neurons. Each column detects one sensory modality. Different modality columns are interspersed.

  1. Layer 4 of each column does not interact with the other columns, but other layers do. Afferent fibers arrive in layer 4 and spread up or down a column. **Layers 1 (most superficial) and 2 are for diffuse, nonspecific input from the lower brain and may control the excitability of a region. Layers 2 and 3 send axons to other cortical areas. Layers 5 and 6 send axons to distant parts of the nervous system. Layer 5 is larger and connects to the brain stem and spinal cord, whereas layer 6 is smaller and connects to the thalamus.**

  2. Neurons stimulate a central area that has increased size with increased signal intensity. All sensory pathways give lateral inhibition to adjacent neurons either through interneurons or by presynaptic inhibition to increase the degree of contrast.

  3. Intensity discrimination decreases as the stimulus intensity increases by overlap. Percent change is more important than total stimulus intensity, so with a greater intensity a larger change is needed to be detected.

4. **Primary somatosensory area** (SS1, Brodmann's area 3, 1, 2)—localizes sensations and detects pressure, weight, shapes (astereognosis), and textures. No pain or temperature loss exists if SS1 is removed, but localization is decreased. The face above the nose has bilateral representation, and the lips have the largest area of representation. Brodmann's area **1** is for rapid adapting skin receptors; **2** is for deep pressure and joint position; **3a** is for muscle, tendon, and joint stretch, located anterior and deep in the central sulcus with connections to the motor cortex; and **3b** is for slowly and rapidly adapting skin receptors. Stimulation elicits contralateral sensory perception.

5. **Secondary somatosensory area** (SS2)—located posterolateral to SS1 on the superior bank of the sylvian fissure. It has poor primary sensory representation but is needed for shape discrimination at least in animals. The lower limbs are located medially. Stimulation elicits **bilateral** sensory perception.

6. **Somatic association areas** (Brodmann's area 5 and 7)—located behind SS1 and above SS2. They have input from SS1, the ventrobasal thalamus (VPL, VPM, posterior thalamic nucleus), visual cortex, and auditory cortex. Stimulation elicits **complex feelings**. A lesion here causes amorphosynthesis (the inability to sense the other side of the body) and **astereognosia**. It is involved with two-point discrimination; in the finger it is 1 mm and in the back it is 30 to 70 mm.

7. Thalamus—can discriminate some touch and much pain and temperature without the cortex. Corticofugal fibers go to peripheral relay nuclei in the thalamus, medulla, and spinal cord to control the sensitivity of a unit, to decrease the lateral spread and increase contrast, and to keep the system in a sensitive range that is not too high or low.

G. Pain and temperature sensation

1. Pain serves a protective function.

2. **Fast pain**—occurs in 0.1 seconds, travels 6 to 30 m/s, and is **sharp** and electric in character. It is carried by **Aδ fibers** and detected by mechanical and thermal receptors in the skin only.

3. **Slow pain**—occurs after 1 second, travels 0.5 to 2 m/s, is slowly increasing, and is **burning**, aching, and throbbing in character. It is carried by **C fibers**, uses all receptors in the skin and deep tissues, and is associated with tissue destruction.

4. Pain receptors—all are free nerve endings located in the skin, periosteum, arterial walls, joint surfaces, and dura. All these respond to mechanical, thermal, and chemical stimuli to different degrees. Very little adaptation exists, and the receptors may even become more sensitive (hyperalgesia) with persistent stimuli. Increased pain intensity is associated with increased tissue damage.

5. Chemicals that excite pain receptors—bradykinin, serotonin, histamine, potassium, acids, ACh, and proteolytic enzymes. Prostaglandins enhance the sensitivity but do not themselves excite the receptors.

6. Thermal pain—starts at 45° C, where tissue damage begins.

7. Tissue ischemia—increases pain by causing altered metabolism of the tissue, possibly by causing increased lactate and acidosis.

8. Spasm of a muscle, artery, or hollow viscus—causes pain by stimulating mechanoreceptors or indirectly closing vessels, causing ischemia (and increasing metabolism so the ischemia is more painful).

9. Pain fibers—enter the spinal cord and ascend or descend one to three segments in **Lissauer's tract** posterior to the dorsal horn before terminating in the dorsal horn.

10. **Neospinothalamic tract**—transmits fast pain. It uses A_δ **fibers** from mechanical and thermal receptors to the DRG (first neuron) lamina 1 (**marginalis**, second neuron), crosses in the anterior commissure, ascends in the anterior lateral tracts to the ventrobasal thalamus (third neuron), and then to the somatosensory cortex (fourth neuron). It has better localization than slow pain but only to approximately 10 cm unless tactile sensation is also stimulated.

11. **Paleospinothalamic tract** transmits slow pain. It uses **C fibers** to laminas 2 and 3 (**substantia gelatinosa**, second neuron) and to lamina 5 by means of interneurons, crosses in the anterior commissure (some remain ipsilateral), go to the reticular formation (third neuron), tectum, and periaqueductal gray, but only 10 to 25% go to the thalamus. The reticular formation then sends fibers to the thalamic intralaminar nuclei, the hypothalamus, and the basal brain for the arousal associated with pain. This system is involved with the suffering aspect of pain. C fibers synapse in the dorsal horn with substance P (slow to build up and slow to be destroyed). It has poor localization to only a limb because of its diffuse projection. One can still have conscious pain even without using the cortex, but the cortex may qualify it.

12. After the destruction of the anterolateral fasciculus, pain returns by polysynaptic pathways.

13. Neurogenic inflammation—caused by an antidromic action potential from the spinal ganglia that releases substance P from the C-fiber terminals in the skin and causes erythema and edema (from increased histamine).

14. The analgesia system

    (a) **periaqueductal gray** and the **periventricular hypothalamus**—contain neurons that send axons releasing enkephalins to the **nucleus raphe magnus** of the lower pons and upper medulla. Secondary neurons send **serotonin**-containing axons to the dorsolateral spinal cord's pain inhibition complex that uses enkephalins for presynaptic pain inhibition (mainly to laminas 1, 2, and 5, the most involved with pain). The neurons in laminas 1 and 5 have presynaptic and postsynaptic opiate receptors. The system blocks pain before it is relayed to the brain. Enkephalin causes presynaptic inhibition of C and Aδ fibers in the dorsal horns by blocking Ca^{++} channels. **NE** from the pons also decreases pain for stress-induced analgesia. Deep brain stimulation of the periventricular and periaqueductal gray has been used to treat chronic pain. **Side effects of**

the periaqueductal gray stimulation are diplopia, oscillopsia, fear, and anxiety. The periventricular gray stimulation is much better tolerated.

(b) Endogenous opiates—β-endorphin (from the hypothalamus and the pituitary), met-enkephalin and leu-enkephalin (in the spinal cord system), and dynorphin (200 times stronger than morphine).

(c) **"Gate control" theory** (introduced by Melzac and Walls in 1965)—large myelinated fibers have a negative dorsal root potential and smaller C fibers have a positive potential. Stimulation of the larger fibers prevents transmission of the pain impulses in the smaller fibers by maintaining a negative potential in the dorsal horns. A problem with this theory is that loss of large myelinated fibers does not produce pain. However, electrical stimulation of large fibers by TENS units, spinal cord stimulators, or deep brain stimulators does appear to cause lateral inhibition of pain. Acupuncture may work by this mechanism, as well as by endogenous opiates and psychogenic input.

15. Referred pain—from visceral pain fibers that synapse in the spinal cord (lamina 5) with the same secondary neurons as the skin so they have a similar central pathway. The only visceral receptors that reach consciousness are for pain.

(a) Visceral pain is different than surface pain because focal injuries are not very painful but diffuse injuries are (i.e., ischemic gut). Pain fibers travel with the sympathetic nerves (occasionally parasympathetic) and are carried only by C fibers.

(b) Visceral pain is caused by ischemia, chemical damage, spasm, distention, and ligamentous stretching. Spasm and distention may cause both mechanical pain and ischemia. The liver parenchyma and alveoli are insensitive to pain, but the bronchi, parietal pleura, liver capsule, and bile ducts are sensitive.

(c) The parietal pleura, peritoneum, and pericardium—supplied by spinal nerves. Referred pain from these areas may cause sharp pain in the wall at a level corresponding to the spinal nerves supplying the viscus.

(d) The heart originated in the neck and upper thorax of the embryo so visceral pain fibers are referred to C3-T5 (neck, shoulder, arm), and the pain is more frequently left-sided than right-sided because left-sided vessels are more often occluded by coronary artery disease.

(e) Pain from viscera may hurt in two locations because of (1) visceral input to sympathetic nerves for referred pain, and (2) parietal irritation input to spinal nerves. Appendicitis typically has (1) periumbilical pain from C fibers, and (2) right lower quadrant pain from Aδ fibers that are more localized when the appendix touches the inflamed peritoneum.

16. Hyperalgia—increased sensitivity (decreased threshold) to pain. It is mediated primarily by increased sensitivity of receptors (sunburn with histamine release) and secondarily by facilitation (spinal cord or thalamic lesion).

17. Hyperpathia—increased reaction to pain, but with increased threshold.

18. Allodynia—pain produced by typically nonpainful stimuli (i.e., light touch).

19. Damaged nerves—may develop axonal sprouts sensitive to EPI or NE, and this may lead to reflex sympathetic dystrophy (RSD).

20. Without normal input, the pain-related neurons in lamina 5 (and later the thalamus) may fire spontaneously and produce phantom pain.

21. Thalamic pain syndrome (Dejerine-Roussy syndrome)—usually due to a posteroventral thalamic stroke with ataxia and contralateral hemianesthesia that in weeks to months has a return of crude sensation but also increased pain and affective unpleasant feelings. It may be caused by the facilitation of the medial thalamic nucleus with increased reticular formation pain transmission.

22. Unlike other sensations, pain is nonadapting.

23. Amitriptyline (Elavil)—helps decrease pain by increasing the serotonin from the descending pathway and increasing NE. NSAIDs decrease the pain-producing protaglandins.

24. Shingles (zoster)—causes pain by irritation of the DRG cells from the virus.

25. Headache—caused by referred pain from deep structures or a sinus, TMJ, ocular structures, dura, or blood vessels. The brain is insensitive to pain, but the sinuses, tentorium, dura, and vessels are sensitive.

　　(a) Supratentorial innervation—by the trigeminal nerve and manifests as frontal head pain. Infratentorial innervation is by C2, CN IX, and CN X and manifests as occipital and retroauricular pain.

　　(b) Postlumbar puncture headache—caused by a decreased CSF volume that allows the weight of the brain to stretch the blood vessels bridging from the surface of the brain to the skull.

　　(c) Migraine headaches—likely a vascular phenomenon caused by reflex spasm of intracranial arteries with ischemia followed by dilation for 24 to 48 hours, with increased blood flow and arterial wall stretching that causes a throbbing headache.

　　(d) Post-ETOH or hangover pain—may be from a chemical irritation to the meninges.

　　(e) Constipation pain—occurs even with a transected spinal cord possibly by absorbed toxins or circulatory system changes.

　　(f) Muscle spasm—produces referred pain over the head.

　　(g) Nasal structures—may become inflamed and cause headache.

　　(h) Eye activity—such as ciliary muscle contraction attempting to obtain focused vision with reflex vasospasm, may cause a retro-orbital headache.

26. Thermal sensation—detected by three receptors:

   (a) Cold receptors—more numerous, and they consist of a myelinated Aδ ending in the basal epidermal cells and also some C free nerve endings.

   (b) Warm receptors—free nerve endings from C fibers and are stimulated if the temperature is $> 30°$ C.

   (c) Pain receptors for extreme temperatures $< 10°$ C and $> 45°$ C. The receptors are in the subcutaneous tissue and are separate from each other. The receptive field is 1 mm in diameter and detects a change in temperature with slow adaptation. It works on receptors by changing the metabolic rate of the neuron. Fibers enter the spinal cord, travel in Lissauer's tract, synapse in laminas 1, 2, and 3 (same as pain), cross to the contralateral side, and ascend to the reticular formation and the ventrobasal thalamus to the SS1 cortex.

VII. VISION

A. Speed of light—in a vacuum it is 300,000 km/s. It is slightly less in air and much less in a liquid or a solid.

B. Refractive index $=$ Velocity in air/velocity in a substance. Refractive index of air $=$ 1. Refraction is the bending of light rays at an interface between substances of different density. It depends on (1) the angle of the interface and the wave front (no refraction if it is perpendicular), and (2) the ratio of the two refractive indices.

C. Convex lens—rays converge at a focal point beyond the lens.

D. Concave lens—rays diverge, with the focal point before the lens.

E. Focal length (f)—determined $1/f = 1/a + 1/b$; a $=$ distance from a point source to the lens; b $=$ distance of focus.

F. Refractive power—increases as the lens bends rays more. It is measured in diopters $=$ 1 m/f. $+$ 1 D means the focal point is 1 m beyond a convex lens, $+$ 2 is 0.5 m, and $+$ 10 is 0.1 m. With a concave lens the diopter number is negative.

G. The eye functions as a camera with four refractive indices: Air/cornea, cornea/aqueous humor, aqueous humor/lens, and lens/vitreous humor. Most refraction is at the air/cornea interface because all the other components are fairly similar in density. The lens is less effective because it is surrounded by fluid, but it is needed for accommodation. The image on the retina is inverted and reversed. The eye unit has a maximum refraction of 59 D. The refractive power in children ranges from 20 to 34 D, with an accommodation of 14 D.

H. Lens—a strong elastic capsule filled with proteinaceous transparent fibers. **When it is relaxed, it has a spherical shape.** Seventy ligaments (zonules) are radially attached to the lens and the ciliary body at the anterior border of the choroid and provide **constant tension** to **keep the lens in a flat shape**.

   (a) **Ciliary body**—has ciliary muscles with two sets of fibers: **Meridional fibers** that attach to the corneoscleral junction and **circular fibers** that are sphincter-like around the eye.

(b) Ciliary muscle contraction—causes the eyeball to become **more narrow** and thus **decreases tension** on the lens and allows it to become more spherical. When the ciliary muscle relaxes, the lens is pulled flat. The **ciliary muscle** is innervated by **parasympathetic nerves** and serves to increase the eye's refractive power for **accommodation** to focus on a closer object.

I. Presbyopia—a condition with a nonaccommodating eye that is permanently focused at a certain distance. Bifocals are needed for near and far clarity. With advancing age, the lens becomes larger, thicker, and less elastic. At 45 years of age only 2 D of change is present, and at 70 years usually no change is present.

J. **Hyperopia** (farsightedness)—caused by either a short eyeball or a weak lens that does not curve enough when the ciliary body is relaxed (the ciliary muscle is contracted). Near vision is difficult. It is treated with a convex lens.

K. **Myopia** (nearsightedness)—caused by either an eyeball that is too long or a lens that is too strong. Light focuses in front of the retina because the lens is unable to straighten enough despite a relaxed ciliary muscle. Far vision is difficult, and it is treated with divergent rays by a concave spherical lens.

L. Astigmatism—caused by refractive error of the lens system from an oblong cornea (rarely from the lens). Rays focus at one distance in one plane and another in another plane. It is treated with spherical and cylindrical lenses of a certain axis.

M. **Cataracts**—opacities of the lens caused by denatured proteins that coagulate. They can be treated by lens removal.

N. When the pupil is small, the eye's focus is better because most of the light enters at a fairly straight trajectory and less refraction is needed.

O. Depth perception—achieved by (1) subconsciously calculating the size of an object visualized against the expected size, (2) moving paralax—closer things move more in a visual field when the head is turned, and (3) stereoptosis—binocular vision with an image hitting different places on each retina (this does not help for objects $>$ 200 ft away).

P. Eye fluid—keeps the eye distended. **Vitreous humor** is a gelatinous mass held by a fibrillary network of proteoglycans. No flow occurs here, but some diffusion occurs. **Aqueous humor** is free flowing, and it is formed and resorbed to regulate intraocular pressure. The ciliary body's ciliary processes secrete the aqueous humor by active Na^+ secretion that pulls in Cl^-, HCO_3^-, and H_2O. The aqueous humor fluid flows out of the pupil and through small trabeculae at the iris-corneal junction and through the **Schlemm's canal** to the venous system.

Q. Intraocular pressure—normally 12 to 20 mm Hg. A tonometer works by a plunger resting on the eye and displacing it a certain distance with a certain pressure.

R. **Glaucoma**—caused by increased intraocular pressure. Levels of 60 to 70 mm Hg commonly cause blindness, although even levels slightly $>$ 20 mm Hg may cause blindness. The elevated pressure on the optic disc causes atrophy. Trabecular aqueous humor outflow decreases with acute inflammation or chronic fibrosis. It is treated with drops to decrease aqueous humor formation or increase its absorption. It can also be treated by surgery to open the pathway.

S. Eye layers—the sclera, choroid (vascular layer), and retina.

T. **Retina**—composed of an outer pigment layer, a layer of rods and cones, an outer limiting membrane, outer nuclear layer (containing cell bodies of the rods and cones), outer plexiform layer, inner nuclear layer, inner plexiform layer, ganglionic layer, optic nerve fiber layer, and inner limiting membrane. The outer pigment layer contains black melanin to prevent light reflection and stores large quantities of vitamin A for exchange with the rods and cones. It is absent in albinism, causing those affected to have poor visual acuity.

U. Retinal detachment—when the retina separates from the pigment epithelium. It occurs with trauma as blood or fluid accumulates behind it or by contractures of fine collagen fibrils in the vitreous humor pulling it unevenly. The retina can maintain its own blood supply for a few days until surgical repair, but if it is delayed longer, it will degenerate and never regain function.

V. **Retinal blood supply**—the inner layers are supplied by the **central retinal artery** that enters through the optic nerve; the outer layers are adherent to the choroid and are fed by **diffusion from the choroid** to the outer segments of the rods and cones.

W. **Macula**—the region of the retina with the highest visual acuity and is < 1 mm^2. The **fovea** is an area of about 0.4 mm in diameter in the center of the macula that contains **only cones**, with the inner layers moved aside for better vision.

X. **Rods**—have an outer segment containing the light-sensitive photochemical rhodopsin with transmembrane proteins and multiple membrane folds shaped into disks. Cones contain other photochemicals.

Y. **Rhodopsin** = scotopsin + 11-cis-retinal. When light energy is absorbed, rhodopsin decomposes by photoactivation of an electron in the retinal component and it changes to the trans form and pulls away from the scotopsin. Rhodopsin + light → bathothodopsin → lumirhodopsin → metarhodopsin 1 → metarhodopsin 2 → scotopsin and all-trans-retinal.

Z. Phototransduction—occurs as activated rhodopsin (metarhodopsin 2) activates a **G protein** that converts **cGMP to 5′ GMP** by cGMP phosphodiesterase and thus **decreases the concentration of cGMP**. This causes a **decreased current** through the cGMP-activated Na$^+$ channels and **hyperpolarization**. Each G protein is regulated by many receptors and regulates many effectors. The **α-subunit binds GTP**, the β and γ subunits hold the α-subunit to the plasma membrane and modulate the GTP/GDP exchange. The conversion from GTP to GDP inactivates the G protein. The **β and γ subunits stabilize the binding of GDP and inhibits the binding of GTP to inactivate the G protein**. When it is activated, the α-subunit has decreased affinity for the β- and γ-subunits. Activation of any G protein inhibits the others in the membrane. Rhodopsin is reformed by all-trans-retinal → 2-cis-retinal + scotopsin → rhodopsin. It is also reformed by all-trans-retinal → all-trans-retinol (vitamin A) → 2-cis-retinol → 2-cis-retinal. Vitamin A is contained in the cytoplasm of rods and the pigment layer of the retina. Extra light-sensitive pigment retinal can be converted to vitamin A for storage.

AA. **Rod receptor potential—hyperpolarizing** because of the **decreased Na^+ conductance** in the outer segment of the rod when the rhodopsin decomposes. Resting membrane potential is -40 mV because of the outer portion being leaky to Na^+, whereas the inner segment pumps it out. The activated membrane potential is -80 mV. Light only has to activate the receptor for 0.0001 ms, but the receptor potential lasts longer than 1 second. The receptor potential is proportional to the light intensity. There is a cascade so one photon of light causes the movement of millions of Na^+ ions. Rhodopsin kinase inactivates the rhodopsin in a fraction of a second. Cones are 300 times less sensitive than rods, so color vision is poor in dim lighting.

BB. Night blindness—due to a severe vitamin A deficiency, in which not enough photosensitive pigment is present to detect less light. This can be cured in 1 hour with IV vitamin A.

CC. Sensitivity of rods and cones—proportional to the opsin concentration. If one is in bright light for a long time, most of the photochemicals are reduced to retinal and opsins, and the retinal is converted to vitamin A to decrease the sensitivity for adaptation. If one is in the dark for a long time, the number of active photopigments is increased (dark adaptation). Cones adapt first within 10 minutes up to 100 times, but while the rods take 40 minutes to adapt, they can become 25,000 times more or less sensitive. Also, light adaptation occurs by a change in pupillary size (30 times change in sensitivity) and by neural adaptation (few fold change) through decreased firing.

DD. **Color vision**—uses photopsins that are sensitive to **red, green, and blue**, with peak absorptions at specific wavelengths. Color is interpreted by the percent stimulation of each color cone (i.e., orange is red 99, green 42, and blue 0). White light is produced by the equal stimulation of red, green, and blue cones. Color constancy is the phenomenon that the brain can (in some cases) detect an object's natural color even after it undergoes color illumination by another colored light source because it compares with white what the color should be. Color blindness is due to the absence of a single or multiple groups of cones. Red or green color blindness is X-linked; rarely is blue missing. This is tested with color spot charts.

EE. Cone pathway—phylogenetically newer, faster, and uses larger cells and fibers. The cone connects to bipolar cells and then to ganglion cells. The rod pathway connects to a bipolar cell, then to an amacrine cell, and finally to a ganglion cell.

FF. Neurotransmitter of rods and cones—**glutamate** $(+)$. Amacrine cells have five types of neurotransmitters and all are inhibitory.

GG. Retinal cells—conduct signals by **electric conduction**, not action potentials (except ganglion cells). This allows graded conduction of signal strength, with increased light intensity causing greater hyperpolarization.

HH. Retinal cells—100 million rods, 3 million cones, and 1.6 million ganglion cells. Each optic nerve fiber receives imput from approximately 60 rods and 2 cones. Near the fovea, rods and cones are more slender and there are less of them per ganglion cell to increase the visual acuity. No rods are in the fovea. The peripheral retina is more sensitive than the fovea to weak light because the rods are 300 times more sensitive than the cones, and 200 rods give input to each ganglion cell.

II. Photoreceptor cells—connect to bipolar and horizontal cells.

JJ. **Horizontal cells**—transmit signals horizontally in the outer plexiform layers. Afferent fibers are from rods and cones. Efferent fibers are to bipolar cells, with lateral inhibition to increase contrast.

KK. **Bipolar cells**—have afferent fibers from rods, cones, and horizontal cells and send efferent fibers to the inner layer amacrine and ganglion cells. Some impulses depolarize and some hyperpolarize to increase the lateral inhibition.

LL. **Amacrine cells**—afferent fibers from bipolar cells and efferent fibers to ganglion cells and horizontal cells in the inner plexus layer.

MM. **Ganglion cells**—send their axons through the optic nerve. **W cells** make up 40% of the fibers, are small, slow (8 m/s), synapse with rods, supply large fields, and are used for directional and dark vision; **X cells** make up 55%, are medium sized, travel at 14 m/s, supply small fields, synapse with cones, and serve accurate color vision; **Y cells** make up 5%, are the largest and fastest (50 m/s), have wide

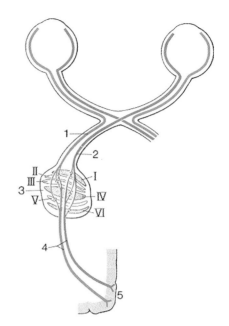

Figure P–1   Visual pathway.

1 Uncrossed fibers from temporal half of retina of left eye
2 Crossed fibers from nasal half of retina of right eye
3 Lateral geniculate body with layers I-VI and projection columns
4 Optic radiation
5 Visual cortex with columns of ocular dominance

fields, and detect changes in fields and black and white vision. There are continuous impulses 5 to 40/s in the background. Ganglion cells respond to borders of vision by excitatory and inhibitory bipolar cells. If light hits all the cells, the stimulation and inhibition cancel each other out so no firing occurs. Each ganglion cell is stimulated by some colors and inhibited by others.

NN. Interplexiform cells—from the inner plexiform layer to the outer plexiform layer and inhibit lateral spread to increase contrast.

OO. Visual pathway's (**Fig. P–1**) optic tract projections

1. **Suprachiasmatic nuclei** of the hypothalamus—for circadian rhythms.

2. **Pretectal nuclei**—for eye and pupillary reflexes.

3. **Superior colliculi**—for conjugate eye movements in response to head movements.

4. **Ventral lateralgeniculate bodies (LGBs)**—to the basal brain for behavioral functions.

5. **Dorsal LGBs (the newest system)**—to relay organized visual fibers to the cortex and gate input (all inhibitory) by corticofugal and midbrain reticular fibers. The LGB layers 1 and 2 contain magnocellular large neurons with input from Y cells and detect black and white vision only. Layers 3 to 6 are parvicellular (smaller cells) and are mostly from the X cells; they transmit color vision. The LGB input is from the **contralateral eye to layers** 1, 4, and 6 and the ipsilateral eye to layers 2, 3, and 5.

PP. Visual cortex

    1. Primary visual cortex or striate cortex—Brodmann's area 17 and is located above and below the calcarine fissure in the medial occipital lobe. The macular field is at the pole with the more peripheral fields located more anteriorly. The upper field is inferior and the right field is on the left.

    2. **Ocular dominance columns**—several million columns with input from alternating eyes that are 40-μm wide and contain approximately 1000 neurons each. No ocular dominance columns exist for the monocular temporal crescent or the blind spot as these are only detected by one eye.

    3. The cortex has six layers. Afferent input from the geniculocalcarine tract is to layer 4, just as in all sensory systems. This layer has thin stripes from alternating eyes that eventually blend together and are called the **lines of Gennari**. The secondary visual area / visual association area (Brodmann's area 18 and 19) is anterior to the primary visual area and is used to analyze visual information.

    4. Cortical processing—there are concentric receptive fields with either on-center or off-center projections from the retinal ganglion cells or the lateral geniculate cells.

        (a) **Simple cells** of the primary visual cortex—have a rectangular field.

        (b) **Complex cells**—have no clear border, and orientation is more important than position.

        (c) **Color blobs**—interspersed among the primary visual columns for color depiction. Threedimensional position, form, and motion are detected in black and white by the Y cells and go to the middle posterior temporal and occipitoparietal cortex. Detail and color go to the inferior ventromedial occipitotemporal cortex.

        (d) Cortex and ganglion cells—have **maximal excitation at the borders of a pattern**. There is serial analysis from simple to complex to hypercomplex cells with increased detail. There is parallel analysis of different information in different places.

QQ. **Blind spot**—15 degrees lateral to central vision and is due to the medial location of the optic disc in the retina.

RR. **Scotoma**—an area of decreased vision surrounded by preserved vision in the visual field. Causes include lead, tobacco, retinal disease, glaucoma, macular degeneration, retinal ischemia, and trauma.

SS. Eye fixation

    1. **Voluntary fixation**—used to locate things and is initiated by the premotor cortex in the **middle frontal gyrus**.

    2. **Involuntary fixation**—used to keep an object in the foveal field and is controlled by the **tertiary visual area (19)**. The eyes have a continuous tremor, a slow drift, and a flicker. The reflex is from area 19 to the superior colliculus to the reticular formation to the extraocular muscle nuclei.

    3. **Saccades**—the eyes jump from one point to the next in a moving field.

4. **Pursuit** movements—keep the eyes fixed on a moving object. Even if the visual cortex is destroyed, the superior colliculus (with visuotopic representation) causes the head to turn toward a visual disturbance by MLF input.

5. **Superior colliculus**—orients the eyes to visual, auditory, or somatic input.

TT. **Strabismus** (cross-eyed)—when no eye fusion is present at birth. It may be horizontal, vertical, or torsional (rotational). One eye may become suppressed and develop decreased acuity.

UU. Parasympathetic innervation to the eye—from the **Edinger-Westphal nucleus** to the third nerve to the ciliary ganglion behind the eye to the **short ciliary nerves** to the ciliary muscle for accommodation and the iris sphincter for miosis.

VV. Sympathetic innervation—from the T1 level to the sympathetic chain to the superior cervical ganglion up along the carotid artery to the small vessels and then as the long and short ciliary nerves to the eye's radial iris fibers for mydriasis, to the **Müller's muscle** of the eyelid, and weakly to the ciliary muscle.

WW. **Accommodation**—by areas 18 and 19 to the pretectal/Edinger-Westphal area to the ciliary muscle.

XX. The pupil is innervated at the iris sphincter by parasympathetics nerves and the radial iris muscles by sympathetic nerves.

YY. **Light reflex**—from the retina to the optic tract to the pretectal nucleus to the Edinger-Westphal nucleus to the third nerve to the iris sphincter. It is decreased with syphilis, ETOH, etc.

ZZ. Accommodation reflex—elicits slight pupillary constriction. If there is no response to light but there is to accommodation, an Argyll Robertson pupil as seen with syphilis is present.

AAA. **Horner's syndrome**—caused by impaired sympathetic input with miosis, ptosis (sympathetic nerves innervate the smooth muscle of the eyelid), anhydrosis, and dilated face vessels.

VIII. HEARING

A. Tympanic membrane—attached to the **malleus**, which is attached to the **incus**, which is attached to the **stapes** that lies against the **oval window** of the cochlea. The malleus handle is constantly pulled inward and tympanic membrane is kept tense by the **tensor tympani muscle** that is innervated by trigeminal branch V3.

B. Ossicles—do not change the amplitude of the sound wave, but they increase the force 1.3 times. Because the surface area of the tympanic membrane is 55 mm^2 and the surface area at the base of the stapes is 3.2 mm^2, the 17 times size change causes a 17 $\times$ 1.3 or a 22 times pressure increase on the cochlea compared with the tympanic membrane.

C. Loud sounds—attenuated by a reflex from the **superior olive**. The tensor tympani muscle (V3) tightens the tympanic membrane and pulls the malleus inward while the **stapedius muscle** (VII) pulls the stapes outward to make a rigid system protecting the cochlea. This masks low-frequency

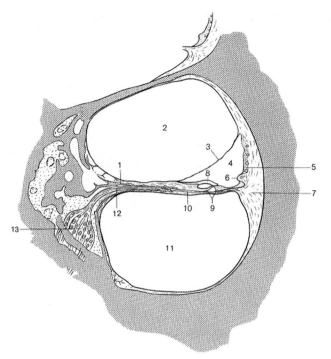

Figure P–2A   Cochlea.

1 Osseous spiral lamina
2 Scala vestibuli
3 Vestibular membrane (Reissner's membrane)
4 Cochlear duct (scala media)
5 Stria vascularis
6 Spiral prominence
7 Spiral ligament
8 Tectorial membrane
9 Spiral organ (of Corti)
10 Basilar membrane
11 Scala tympani
12 Dendrites of cell bodies situated in spiral ganglion of cochlea which pass to sensory (hair) cells of organ of Corti
13 Spiral ganglion of cochlea; axons form the cochlear nerve of vestibulocochlear nerve

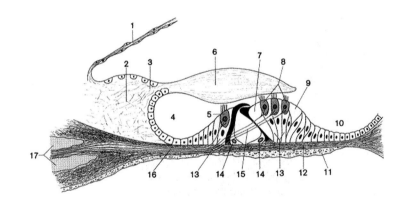

Figure P–2B   Cochlea.

1 Vestibular membrane (Reissner's membrane)
2 Limbus of osseous spiral lamina
3 Vestibular lip
4 Internal spiral sulcus
5 Inner hair (sensory) cell
6 Tectorial membrane
7 Nuel's space
8 Outer hair (sensory) cells
9 Outer tunnel
10 External spiral sulcus
11 Lining tissue of scala tympani
12 Basilar membrane
13 Outer phalangeal (Deiter's) cells
14 Pillar cells
15 Nerve fibers in inner tunnel
16 Dendrites of cell bodies located in spiral ganglion
17 Osseous spiral lamina

sounds in a loud environment and also serves to decrease the hearing of one's own speech (it is activated with speech production).

D. Cochlea (**Fig. P–2A and B**)—consists of three side-by-side coiled tubes that turn 2.5 times with the scala media in the center. The sound vibrations enter the **scala vestibuli** and also the **scala media** because **Reissner's membrane** is flexible. The **basilar membrane** is a fibrous membrane separating the scala media and **scala tympani** and is made of 25,000 fibers extending from the bony center of the cochlea (**modiolus**) to the outer wall. These are reedlike fibers fixed at the modiolus and free at the outer point to enable them to vibrate. Reeds (basilar fibers) get longer and narrower as they approach the apex of the cochlea so they become less stiff. Near the base at the oval window they are stiff, short, and have a higher frequency. **Vibrations at the apex have a lower frequency.** The cochlea is bounded on all sides by bony walls so if the stapes and the oval window move inward, the round window pushes outward, and the basilar reeds move inward. Sound waves proceed forward until they meet the reed with the same frequency, which then vibrates with ease until the sound dies out. High-frequency waves travel only short distances in the cochlea.

E. **Organ of Corti**—the hearing receptor that senses vibration and it is located on the surface of the **basilar membrane**. It has internal and external **hair cells**. The bases and sides of the hair cells synapse with the cochlear nerve endings that have cell bodies in the **spiral ganglion** in the modiolus at the center of the cochlea. Axons from the spiral ganglion make up the cochlear nerve.

1. A hundred stereocilia project from each of the hair cells into the gel of the **tectorial membrane** in the **scala media**. They bend one way to cause hyperpolarization and the other for depolarization. The tectorial membrane remains still while the basilar membrane moves.

2. Depolarization—occurs by increased K^+ conductance into the stereocilia. The scala media contains **endolymph**, whereas the scala vestibuli and the scala tympani contain **perilymph** that communicates with the CSF and the perilymph of the vestibular organs.

3. Endolymph—secreted by the stria vascularis and has **increased K^+ and decreased Na^+** more like intracellular fluid (unlike perilymph). The scala media's endolymph potential is $+80$ mV compared with the perilymph because of the active pumping in of K^+. This creates the **endocochlear potential**.

4. The hair cell's body is in the perilymph and has a potential of -60 mV with respect to the perilymph, whereas the cilia lies in the endolymph where the intracellular potential difference is -140 mV, making the cilia very sensitive.

F. Sound interpretation—involves the **place principle** in which stimulation of different areas in the cochlea causes different nerves to fire and this determines **frequency (pitch)**. The cochlear nucleus can still distinguish different frequencies if part of the cochlea is removed. Loudness is detected by increased amplitude, causing an increased frequency of hair cell firing and spatial summation with more cilia being pulled. Humans are able to distinguish 1 dB change in sound intensity. One can hear high-frequency sounds at low intensity, but low-frequency sounds need higher intensity. Humans' frequency range is from 20 to 20,000 cycles/s (Hz) but below 60 dB only 500 to 5000 cycles/s are able to be detected.

G. Auditory pathway (see Chapter 1)—from the **spiral ganglion** (first neuron) to the dorsal and ventral **cochlear nuclei** (second neuron) to the **trapezoid body** to the ipsilateral and contralateral **superior olivary nucleus** (third neuron) to the **lateral lemniscus** and the nucleus of the lateral lemniscus (fourth neuron) to the **inferior colliculus** (fifth neuron) to the **MGB** (sixth neuron) to the **auditory cortex** (seventh neuron).

1. The fibers from the dorsal cochlear nuclei bypass the superior olivary nucleus and the nucleus of the lateral lemniscus to synapse on the neurons in the inferior colliculus (third neuron). Fibers cross to the contralateral side from the ventral cochlear nuclei by way of the trapezoid body (to the superior olivary nucleus), in the nucleus of the lateral lemniscus by way of the **commissure of Probst**, and in the inferior colliculus by way of the inferior collicular commissure.

2. There is bilateral representation with **slightly greater hearing on the contralateral side**. Crossover pathways render unilateral hearing loss uncommon with lesions in the brain stem or more proximally. There are collateral fibers to the reticular formation, the vermis, and the spinal cord. Tonotopic orientation is maintained in the tracts. **The superior olivary nucleus inhibits the hair cells to isolate out certain sounds.**

H. **Primary auditory cortex** (area 41)—receives afferent fibers from the medial geniculate body. The auditory association area (area 42) receives afferent fibers from the primary auditory cortex and the thalamic association areas. There is **tonotopic organization** by sound frequency and also organization by location. Lateral inhibition sharpens sound detection but decreases the frequency range heard from the cochlea.

1. Cortex—needed for tonal and sequential sound pattern discrimination. If the primary human auditory cortex is destroyed, there is decreased spatial localization because both sides compare the intensity of low-frequency input and the time difference of arrival with high-frequency input. If the secondary auditory cortex is destroyed, there is decreased sensitivity. If the association areas are destroyed, there is sound agnosia.

2. **Localization—also achieved by the medial superior olivary nucleus, which detects the time lag between the ears and by the lateral superior olivary nucleus, which detects the intensity change between the ears.** The elderly lose high-frequency discrimination. Chronic exposure to loud noises such as music and industrial equipment can cause high-frequency hearing loss. Ototoxic medications tend to cause loss of all frequencies.

IX. TASTE

A. Taste—detected by the taste buds and by smell and texture. It functions to help one choose safe and nutritious foods. Deer use salt licks to fill their sodium requirements. The person who has decreased PTH levels craves foods high in calcium. The hypoglycemic individual craves sweets. People develop positive or negative emotions associated with food that made them happy or sick.

B. Taste sensation—there are receptors for Na^+, K^+, Cl^-, adenosine, inosine, glutamate, H^+, sweet, and bitter.

C. Four major taste sensations:

1. Sour—responds to acids, is proportional to H^+ concentration, and is detected on the lateral aspect of the tongue.

2. Salt responds to Na^+ and K^+ and is detected on the tip of the tongue.

3. Sweet—responds to sugar, alcohol, and many organic chemicals, and is detected on the tip of the tongue.

4. Bitter—responds to organic molecules, especially long chains with N and alkaloids (i.e., caffeine, nicotine, quinine, and deadly plant toxins), and is detected on the back of the tongue and palate.

D. Taste buds—made of about 40 epithelial cells consisting of supporting sustentacular cells and taste cells that are constantly remade and replaced with newer or dividing ones at the center. Microvilli project from the cells. Taste nerve fibers are stimulated by the taste receptor cells that are able to detect more than one stimulus. Adults have approximately 10,000 taste buds, but these decrease with age. The taste cell binds a chemical and then depolarizes by increasing Na^+ conductance. The taste is intense at first, but adaptation is quick. The chemical is washed away with saliva.

E. The anterior $\frac{2}{3}$ of the tongue carries sensation by CN V3 (lingual nerve) and taste by CN VII (chorda tympani). The posterior $\frac{1}{3}$ of the tongue is innervated for sensation and taste by CN IX. The base of the tongue and pharynx are innervated by CN X for both sensation and taste. These fibers from CN VII, IX, and X go to the nucleus solitarius (with the fibers from CN VII being most rostral) and then to the thalamic VPM nucleus and then to the cortex.

F. Reflexes are from the solitary tract to the superior and inferior salivatory nuclei.

G. Most sensory systems adapt at the receptors, but taste has 50% adaptation at the receptors and 50% in CNS.

X. SMELL

A. Seven known olfactory stimulants—camphoraceous, musky, pungent, putrid, floral, peppermint, and ethereal. There may be many more.

B. Many people cannot detect certain odors because they are missing a receptor.

C. An affective component of smell can alter sex drive and appetite.

D. Only a small range of intensity is detected. It is apparently more important that the smell is present than how much is present.

E. Olfactory membrane—located in the superior nasal cavity. The **olfactory cells** are bipolar cells from the CNS (approximately 100 million) that are embedded in the olfactory epithelium and are supported by sustentacular cells. The mucosal surface of the cell has 6 to 12 olfactory hairs or cilia projecting into the mucus secreted by **Bowman's glands**. The cilia have odor-binding proteins projecting through their membranes that may sense smell by changing ion flow or by cAMP formation. Detected substances must be volatile and may be water (mucus) or lipid (membrane) soluble.

F. The RMP is −55 mV and there is continuous firing. Stimulation increases the action potential rate in proportion to the stimulus strength. Adaptation of 50% occurs in 1 second and then continues gradually to baseline. Adaptation is at the level of the granule cells (inhibitory) in the olfactory bulb.

G. The olfactory bulb lies over the cribriform plate. Axons from the olfactory cells (first neuron) go to the glomeruli in the olfactory bulb (second neuron). There are 25,000 axons per **glomerulus**, which is composed of 25 **mitral cells** and 60 **tufted cells**. The glomeruli send axons to the CNS by way of a tract (CN 1) and are tonically active with specific glomeruli detecting specific smells. The olfactory tract divides into **medial and lateral olfactory stria** that travel to medial and lateral olfactory areas. The **medial olfactory area** contains the septal nuclei anterior and superior to the hypothalamus. It is phylogenetically old and is used for primary reflexes such as salivation, licking, and emotion. The **lateral olfactory area** is in the prepyriform and **pyriform cortex** and the cortex over the amygdala nucleus. It has efferents to the limbic system but especially the hippocampus, creating a strong association between smell and memory. This correlates with absolute aversion to foods with prior nausea and vomiting by learning. These are old areas with paleocortex. The newest olfactory area includes the DM thalamus that connects to the posterolateral orbitofrontal cortex for conscious analysis of odor.

H. Smell is the only sensation not connected directly to the thalamus (with the exception of the phylogenetically recent component).

I. The cortex sends impulses to the **granule cells** to inhibit the mitral and tufted cells to possibly sharpen the distinction of smells.

XI. MOTOR SYSTEMS

A. Topographical representation—in the vermis and the intermediate zone of the cerebellum, the sensory and motor cortex, the basal ganglia, the red nucleus, and the reticular formation.

B. The spinal cord has many preset activities that the brain modulates. The walking reflex is contained in the spinal cord, so animals can still walk after the cervical cord is cut. The decerebrate animal is cut at the lower midbrain so there is no longer inhibition of the pontine reticular formation's and the vestibular nucleus' inputs.

C. Sensory fibers send a branch to the spinal gray matter for reflexes.

D. There are many thousand anterior motor neurons per spinal level.

1. **Alpha motor neurons**—larger and innervate skeletal muscle by sending Aα fibers to the large skeletal muscle fibers in the motor unit.

2. **Gamma motor neurons**—smaller, 50% less numerous, and send Aδ fibers to the intrafusal fibers of the muscle spindle. The interneurons are smaller, very excitable, and have many connections.

3. **Almost all of the corticospinal tract fibers synapse first on interneurons.** Very few sensory axons synapse directly on anterior motor neurons.

E. **Renshaw cells**—in the anterior horn. An alpha motor neuron's axon sends a branch to a Renshaw cell, which uses the neurotransmitter **glycine** to inhibit the surrounding alpha motor neuron synergists and inhibit the antagonist's inhibitors to create a negative feedback loop that sharpens signals in a manner similar to lateral inhibition.

F. Propriospinal fibers—connect various spinal cord segments and make up more than 50% of the spinal cord fibers.

G. Feedback during movement —obtained by the muscle spindles and the Golgi tendon organs.

H. **Muscle spindle**—located in the belly of the muscle and detects **length and velocity of change in length** of the muscle. It is stimulated by the stretching of the midportion of the spindle and increases firing with muscle stretch and decreases firing with muscle contraction.

1. It is in **parallel** with the muscle fibers and is composed of 3 to 12 intrafusal muscle fibers attached to the large extrafusal fibers. The central part is without actin and myosin so it does not contract. The ends have gamma motor neuron input. The spindle output is sensory.

2. **Primary ending (annulospiral ending)—a Ia fiber**, circles the center of the muscle fiber, travels at 70 to 120 m/s, and is the fastest sensory fiber in the body. The **secondary ending (flower-spray ending) is a II fiber**, is on one end of a primary ending, and travels more slowly.

3. Intrafusal fibers—**the nuclear bag fibers, which are innervated by the primary sensory ending** and **the nuclear chain fibers, which are smaller and innervated by the primary and secondary sensory endings**.

4. Impulses are proportional to the degree of stretching. The static response is transmitted by the nuclear chain fibers that fire tonically when the muscle is stretched. The dynamic response is by the nuclear bag fibers and detects the rate of change with tonic firing at a baseline rate that increases or decreases with an increased or decreased rate of stretch.

5. Myotactic (muscle stretch) reflex—when a muscle is stretched, the impulse travels from the spindle's Ia fibers to the alpha motor neuron that causes contraction by a **monosynaptic reflex**. The damping mechanism smoothes contractions from multiple sources so the movement is not jerky.

6. Thirty-one percent of motor nerve fibers are from gamma motor neurons. There is coactivation as the gamma motor neuron is stimulated at the same time as the alpha motor neuron to keep it under the same load and so that it does not oppose the initial contraction.

7. Servo-assist mechanism—works during a contraction against a load where the intrafusal fibers get shorter than the extrafusal fibers. This causes a reflex increase in the muscle activity so the contraction becomes less load sensitive.

8. Gamma motor neurons—innervated by the bulboreticular facilitory region, the cerebellum, the basal ganglia, and the cortex. Gamma motor neurons have decreased activity with cerebellar lesions so there is decreased tone.

9. Stretch reflex—demonstrates tone to evaluate the brain's input to the spinal cord. The cortex inhibits the reflex, whereas the brain stem increases it. Damage to the cortex causes hyperreflexia, whereas damage to the brain stem causes hyporeflexia.

10. Clonus—an oscillation of the muscle jerk response from the intermittent stretch on the spindle against force. It is increased if the reflex is sensitized by facilitory impulses in the brain (especially decerebrate).

I. **Golgi tendon organs**—encapsulated receptors with bundles of tendon fibers passing through them at the muscle-tendon junction. There are 10 to 15 muscle fibers per tendon organ, and they detect the tension of the muscle fiber. They increase their firing rate with **active contraction and passive stretch**. The afferent signal is carried by **Ib fibers** to interneurons that decrease the alpha motor neuron output (also to the cortex and spinocerebellar tracts). The reflex is **not monosynaptic**. It prevents muscle tearing and serves to equalize the force in the muscle so the fibers with too much tension can relax.

J. The **dorsal spinocerebellar tracts**—carry information from the muscle spindles and the Golgi tendon organs at speeds as fast as **120 m/s**. Fibers also go to the reticular formation and the cortex.

K. Many reflexes are stored in the spinal cord:

1. Flexor (withdrawal) reflex—seen in spinal or decerebrate animals. This occurs when a stimulus on a limb elicits withdrawal. It is evoked more by pain than touch and uses interneurons with divergence and reciprocal inhibition of antagonists and circuits to prolong the discharge after the stimulus has gone. There is a longer duration with an increased signal intensity and it may last 1 to 3 seconds.

2. Crossed extensor reflex—when the opposite limb extends 0.2 to 0.5 seconds after the flexor reflex to push the body from the stimulus and is mediated by interneurons.

3. Positive supportive reaction—when pressure on the footpad of a spinal or decerebrate animal causes limb extension and standing.

4. Cord righting reflex—enables a spinal animal to move to stand up.

5. Rhythmic stepping reflex—when the limb flexes and then extends. This is controlled by oscillating circuits with reciprocal inhibition of agonists and antagonists. It does not need sensory input, but sensation does increase and decrease the rate.

6. Rhythmic walking reflex—enables the two sides of the spinal cord to coordinate both limbs.

7. Rhythmic galloping reflex—allows both front and back legs to move together.

8. Scratch reflex—triggered by itch and tickle.

L. Muscle spasm—a response to pain. It is decreased with analgesics or antispasmodics. A cramp is a reflex contraction by pain, cold, or decreased blood flow and is treated with reciprocal inhibition by contracting antagonist muscles.

M. Autonomic reflexes—change the vascular tone to control body temperature, cause sweating, and control blood pressure. Peritoneo-intestinal reflexes decrease gut motility with peritoneal irritation. Evacuation reflexes exist for the bladder and colon. The mass reflex in the spinal animal occurs when strong pain or increased filling of the bladder or gut may cause body flexor spasms, evacuation of the colon and bladder, increased blood pressure, and sweating. It may be considered to be a spinal cord seizure.

N. **Spinal shock**—when all function and all reflexes of the spinal cord are lost after injury. The spinal cord is normally under tonic stimulation from the corticospinal tracts, the reticulospinal tracts, and the vestibulospinal tracts. After transection, within hours to weeks, the spinal neurons regain partial excitability. There is an immediate decrease in blood pressure to 80 mm Hg (because of the absence of sympathetic tone and loss of skeletal muscle reflexes). The first reflexes to return are the stretch reflexes (bulbocavernosus reflex) followed by others. The **bulbocavernosus reflex** may return within hours of injury. More complex reflexes may take weeks. Extracellular hyperkalemia in the spinal cord is believed to be an important cause of spinal shock.

O. **Primary motor cortex**—Brodmann's area 4. The homunculus was mapped by Penfield and Rasmussen and $>50\%$ is dedicated to hand and face function. **Betz's cells** are large pyramidal neurons, are only in the primary motor cortex, send impulses at speeds of 70 m/s (the fastest fibers from the brain to the spinal cord), and make up **3%** of corticospinal tract (34,000 of the million fibers in each corticospinal tract).

   1. Efferent fibers from the motor cortex—also include collateral fibers to the cortex (for lateral inhibition), fibers to the caudate and putamen, the red nucleus (rubrospinal), the reticular formation (reticulospinal and cerebellar), the vestibular system (vestibulospinal and cerebellar), and the inferior olive (olivocerebellar).

   2. Afferent fibers—somatosensory input (muscle spindles with positive feedback if they move more than extrafusal fibers), visual cortex, auditory cortex, frontal cortex, contralateral motor cortex by way of the corpus callosum, the ventrobasal thalamus (somatosensory), the VL and VA thalamus (with input from the cerebellum and basal ganglia), and the intralaminar nuclei of the thalamus (for level of excitability).

   3. It is arranged in vertical columns: Layers 2 to 4 for input, **layer 5 with Betz's cells** for long output, and layer 6 for intracortical output. Fifty to 100 Betz's cells are needed to contract one muscle. Dynamic neurons develop force and static neurons maintain it.

P. **Premotor area**—**Brodmann's area 6 and** is located anterior to area 4. It has the same layered organization as area 4 and contains patterns for specific tasks. The circuit is from the premotor cortex to the basal ganglia to the thalamus to area 4.

   1. **Broca's area (area 44)**—in the posterior inferior frontal gyrus and functions in choosing correct words and coordinating breathing with voice.

   2. The **frontal eye field (area 8)**—located just above Broca's area in the middle frontal gyrus and controls eyelid movements (blinking) and horizontal saccadic eye movements to the opposite side. If it is damaged, one can still lock in on targets by occipital cortical function.

3. Head rotation area—just above the eye field and functions to turn the head with eye movements.

4. Hand skill area—just above the head rotation area and is anterior to the primary motor hand area. A lesion here causes motor apraxia.

Q. **Supplemental motor area (area 6)**—located anterior and superior to the premotor cortex. It is mainly along the medial side of the hemisphere adjacent to the longitudinal fissure with a little extension over the superior surface of the hemisphere. The **lower limb area is posterior and the face area is anterior**. This cortex requires a stronger stimulus to elicit contraction than other areas, and stimulation elicits **bilateral contractions**. It serves to set complex actions that serve as a background for finer actions. Injury causes decreased voluntary movement and speech output that usually resolves in 6 weeks.

R. Corticospinal tract (pyramidal tract)—contains 1 million fibers, **30% from area 4, 30% from the premotor (area 6) and supplementary motor cortices, and 40% sensory fibers**. It travels in the **posterior limb** of the IC and most fibers cross to the **contralateral corticospinal tract** to end on interneurons (few go to sensory relays or alpha motor neurons). The **ventral corticospinal tract** is mainly **ipsilateral**, but many fibers cross at lower levels in the spinal cord. Its fibers are mainly from the supplementary motor cortex and are used for **posture control**.

S. Red nucleus—functions like the corticospinal tract to the distal limbs but is less fine and serves as an accessory route of corticospinal transmission when the corticospinal tract is destroyed. It has afferent input from corticospinal branches and corticorubral fibers to a magnocellular area with large Betz-like neurons. The efferent fibers are in the rubrospinal tract that crosses just anterior to the corticospinal tract. There is also afferent input from the dentate and interposed nuclei and efferent fibers to the interposed nucleus. It is also connected to the reticular formation. There is **somatotopic organization**.

T. **Lateral motor system** of the spinal cord—includes the corticospinal tract and the rubrospinal tract. They have increased direct connections with alpha motor neurons in the cervical cord for fine motor control of the hand.

1. The spinal cord helps to grade power with the servo-assist mechanism. The spinal cord has reciprocal antagonist reflexes so the brain only needs to make simple commands for a complex task.

2. If the primary motor cortex is removed, there are no voluntary fine movements of the hand and there is decreased tone because the corticospinal tract normally provides tonic excitatory input to the spinal cord.

3. Damage to the basal ganglia, deep structures, and adjacent cortex causes increased tone because the tonic inhibition to the vestibular system and the reticular formation is removed.

4. The Babinski response is present only if there is damage to the corticospinal tract or the primary motor cortex. The corticospinal tract is the phylogenetically recent system, delivers fine control,

and overrides the more primitive systems such as the rubrospinal system. The noncorticospinal tracts are older systems and are used for pain avoidance by withdrawal mechanisms. When the corticospinal system is damaged, the older systems take over.

U. Medial motor system of the spinal cord—includes the vestibulospinal and reticulospinal tracts to the axial and limb-girdle muscles.

1. **Pontine reticular nucleus**—laterally situated, extends up to the midbrain, and excites antigravity muscles by way of the lateral reticulospinal tract to the medial anterior horn cells. It is stimulated by the vestibular nucleus and the cerebellum.

2. **Medullary reticular nucleus**—ventromedial and inhibits antigravity muscles by means of the medial reticulospinal tract (lateral fibers). It is stimulated by the corticospinal and rubrospinal tracts and other motor groups.

3. **Vestibular nucleus**—stimulates antigravity muscles to maintain equilibrium (with the help of the pontine reticular formation). The lateral vestibular nucleus sends fibers to the **lateral and medial vestibulospinal tracts**.

V. **Decerebrate rigidity**—caused by sectioning the brain stem between the pons and the midbrain. There is increased antigravity muscle action of the neck, trunk, and lower limb muscles. **This lesion blocks the normal stimulatory input to medullary reticular formation from the cortex, red nucleus, and basal ganglia.** This allows the pontine reticular nucleus and lateral vestibular nucleus to take over with increased and unopposed antigravity tone.

1. The increased **spasticity** (resistance to change in muscle length) is by increased **gamma motor neuron** stimulation compared with alpha motor neuron stimulation from the pontine reticular nucleus and the vestibular nucleus. This increased tone can therefore be abolished by sectioning the dorsal spinal roots and abolishing the δ loop (α rigidity).

2. If the anterior lobe of the cerebellum is destroyed, there is no longer Purkinje's cell–mediated inhibition of the lateral vestibular nucleus, and this causes increased extensor tone.

W. **Spasticity**—characterized by unidirectional resistance to change, velocity dependency, and increased reflexes. **Rigidity** has bidirectional resistance to change, is not velocity dependent, and is not associated with hyperreflexia. Cerebellar spasticity is not dependent on gamma motor neurons, so it is not alleviated with posterior root sectioning. Refer to Chapter 4 for more information about spasticity and rigidity.

XII. VESTIBULAR SYSTEM (FIG. P–3)

A. The bony labyrinth surrounds the membranous labyrinth.

B. **Macula**—the sensory organ of the **utricle and the saccule**. It contains hair cells with cilia that are embedded in a gelatinous layer containing calcium carbonate **otoliths**. The hair cells synapse with the

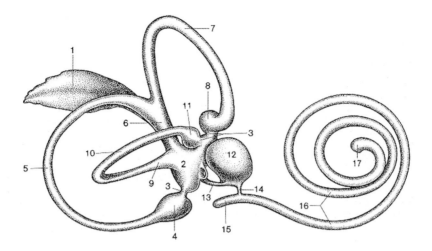

Figure P–3   Membranous labyrinth.

1 Endolymphatic sac
2 Utricle
3 Ampullary crus (of each semicircular duct)
4 Ampulla of posterior semicircular duct
5 Posterior semicircular duct
6 Common crus (of posterior and anterior semicircular
   ducts)
7 Anterior semicircular duct

8 Ampulla of anterior semicircular duct
9 Simple crus of lateral semicircular duct
10 Lateral semicircular duct
11 Ampulla of lateral semicircular duct
12 Saccule
13 Utriculosaccular duct
14 Ductus reuniens
15 Vestibular cecum
16 Cochlear duct
17 Cupolar cecum

vestibular nerve. Each hair cell has 50 to 70 stereocilia and one large kinocilium. All cilia are connected at the tip in the gel layer and become gradually longer until they reach the kinocilium. When they bend toward the kinocilium, there is increased Na^+ conductance causing depolarization. When they bend away, there is decreased Na^+ conductance causing hyperpolarization. There is a baseline firing rate of 100 impulses/s that may increase to many hundred or decrease to 0. The hair cells face various directions, so some depolarize with forward bending, whereas others do for backward or lateral bending.

C. **Utricle**—has its **macula** on the horizontal plane. It senses the direction of gravitational or accelerative forces when one is **upright**, and it is less effective as the head moves from vertical.

D. **Saccule**—has its **macula** vertical so it functions when one is horizontal or **supine**.

E. Three **semicircular canals** (anterior, posterior, and horizontal)—at right angles to each other so they can detect motion in any of three planes. If the head is bent forward from the horizontal 30 degrees, the horizontal canal is horizontal with the earth's surface, the anterior canal is forward and 45 degrees lateral, and the posterior canal is backward and 45 degrees lateral.

F. **Ampulla**—a dilation at the end of each semicircular canal that is filled with **endolymph**. It contains the **crista ampullaris**, the sensory organ of the semicircular canals, which has hair cells with cilia that project into the gel cup (cupula). There is increased or decreased Na^+ conductance altered by the direction of the bending. The rate of the action potential is proportional to the direction of the rotation. With head rotation, the fluid remains stationary, but the semicircular canal moves and bends the hair cell's cilia in the **cupula**. Rotation to the left causes the cilia to bend to the right.

G. Macula—detects **static and linear acceleration** (but not velocity) because when the head moves forward, otoliths relatively move backward because they have more inertia than the surrounding fluid. The semicircular canals detect **angular acceleration** because fluid in the ducts stay still from inertia despite head movement. The semicircular canals predict a fall by detecting head rotation so an early adjustment can be made, whereas the utricle only acts after the falling has begun. If the flocculonodular lobe is removed, impaired function of the semicircular canals but not the macula occurs.

H. Posture reflex—anticipates a balance change and elicits a spinal reflex to stay standing. The semicircular ducts cause the eyes to move in a direction equal and opposite to the head by means of the MLF. The vestibular apparatus only detects head movements, whereas the orientation of the head against the neck and the body is detected by proprioception input to the vestibular system, the reticular formation, and the cerebellum. Vision can elicit an equilibrium response without the vestibular system.

I. The vestibular nerve goes to the vestibular nucleus and also to the cerebellum, which connects to the reticular formation and the spinal cord. The flocculonodular lobe functions with the semicircular canals to detect rapid changes in direction. The uvula maintains static equilibrium. The cerebellum and vestibular system gives input to the MLF for eye movement and to the primary equilibrium cortex in the parietal lobe deep in the sylvian fissure opposite the auditory cortex of the superior temporal gyrus.

J. **Superior and medial vestibular nuclei**—involved with eye reflexes. They receive afferent input from the semicircular canals and have efferent fibers to the MLF for eye movement and to the medial vestibulospinal tract for head and neck movement. The **medial vestibular nucleus** is the largest vestibular nucleus and sends crossed fibers to all extraocular nerve nuclei and to the cerebellum. The **superior vestibular nucleus** sends uncrossed fibers by way of the MLF to the CN III and IV nuclei.

K. **Lateral vestibular nucleus (Deiter's nucleus)**—involved with posture. It has afferent fibers from the utricle (from the superior vestibular ganglion) and the saccule (from the inferior vestibular ganglion) and efferent fibers to the lateral vestibulospinal tract that serve to elicit lower limb extension and upper limb flexion for posture control. It stimulates both alpha and gamma motor neurons and is tonically inhibited by Purkinje's cells so that removal of the anterior lobe of the cerebellum causes spasticity.

L. **Inferior vestibular nucleus**—integrates input from the vestibular system and the cerebellum. It has afferent input from the semicircular canals and the utricle and efferent fibers to the cerebellum and the reticular formation.

M. Stereotyped body movements—stored in various parts of the CNS. Forward flexion, extension, and rotation are in the midbrain and lower thalamus. Rotational eye movement and head movement is by the interstitial nucleus of the midbrain near the MLF. Raising of the head and the body is in the prestitial nucleus at the junction of the midbrain and the thalamus. Flexion of the head and the body is at the nucleus precommissuralis at the level of the posterior commissure. Turning of the body is at the pontine and midbrain reticular formation.

XIII. CEREBELLUM

A. Cerebellum—controls the timing of motor movements and the rapid progression of agonist/antagonist interplay. It sequences and corrects activities, compares intention with action by means of sensory input, and aids the cortex in planning the next movement. It may have memory to learn by mistakes. Stimulation elicits no motor or sensory activity.

B. **Vermis**—involved with the axial body (neck, shoulders, and hips). It has afferent input from the motor cortex, brain stem and spinal cord. Efferent fibers go to the motor cortex, red nucleus, and reticular formation.

C. **Intermediate zone**—controls the distal limbs. It has similar afferent and efferent connections as the vermis.

D. **Lateral zone**—involved with the planning of sequential motor movements. There is **no known topographic representation**. It is connected to the association areas of the cortex (premotor, somatic, and somatic association).

E. Afferent tracts

   1. **Inferior cerebellar peduncle**

      (a) **Juxtarestiform body**
         (i)   **Vestibulocerebellar**—vestibular nucleus to the fastigial nucleus of the flocculonodular lobe.

      (b) **Restiform body**
         (i)   **Olivocerebellar**—motor cortex, basal ganglia, reticular formation, and spinal cord to the inferior olive to the cerebellum.
         (ii) **Reticulocerebellar**—reticular nucleus to the vermis.
         (iii) **Dorsal spinocerebellar**—from the muscle spindles, Golgi tendon organs, tactile, and joint receptors to **Clarke's column** to the dorsospinalcerebellar tract up the inferior peduncle to the ipsilateral vermis and the intermediate zone. The spinocerebellar tracts conduct impulses at 120 m/s and are the fastest fibers in the central nervous system.

   2. **Middle cerebellar peduncle: Corticopontocerebellar**—from the motor, premotor, and sensory cortices to the pontine nucleus to the contralateral cerebellar hemisphere.

   3. **Superior cerebellar peduncle: Ventral spinocerebellar**—from the anterior motor neurons through the superior peduncle to the bilateral cerebellum as an efference copy telling the cerebellum what motor signals are received in the spinal cord from the corticospinal tracts and the rubrospinal tracts.

   4. Deep nuclear input—from both the cortex and the sensory afferent tracts.

   5. Incoming fibers to the cerebellum divide with one fiber going to the deep nuclei and one to the cortex.

F. Efferent tracts

   1. **Inferior cerebellar peduncle** (by way of the **juxtarestiform body**)

     (a) Flocculonodular lobe to the lateral vestibular nucleus (lesion causes nystagmus).

     (b) Vermis to the fastigial nucleus to the pons and medulla for equilibrium and posture (lesion causes truncal ataxia and scanning speech).

   2. **Superior cerebellar peduncle**

     (a) Intermediate zone to the **interposed nuclei** to the VL and VPLo thalamus to the cortex, thalamus, basal ganglia, red nucleus (mainly), and midbrain reticular formation for distal limb agonist/antagonist control (lesion causes appendicular ataxia).

     (b) Lateral zone to the **dentate nucleus** to the VL and VPLo thalamus to the cortex (area 4) for coordination of sequential action (lesion causes intention tremor).

   3. There is decreased tone with injury to the vermis or intermediate zone.

G. The cerebellum has 30 million functional units, each centered around a Purkinje's cell. The cortex has a **molecular layer** (with basket and stellate cells), a **Purkinje's layer**, and a **granular layer** (with granule and Golgi's type II cells). All the cells are inhibitory except the granule cells. The output of the functional unit is to the cells of the deep nuclei (these are excitatory) that are inhibited by Purkinje's cells and excited by the peripheral afferents (the climbing and mossy fibers).

   1. **Climbing fibers** (excitatory)—from the inferior olivary complex to the Purkinje's cells and the deep nuclear cells. One fiber stimulates 10 Purkinje's cells with 300 synapses in the molecular layer and one fiber also stimulates multiple deep nuclear cells, but the strongest input is to the Purkinje's cells.

   2. **Mossy fibers** (excitatory)—from all the other afferent sources (cortex, brain stem, spinal cord, etc.) to the deep nuclear cells and to the granular layer with synapses on hundreds of granule cells to form glomeruli.

   3. **Granule cells** (excitatory, glutamate is the neurotransmitter)—project to the molecular layer where the axon bifurcates and forms **parallel nerve fibers** that travel parallel to the axis of the foliae. They form 80,000 to 200,000 synapses with each Purkinje's cell. Each fiber contacts 250 to 500 Purkinje's cells. There are 500 to 1000 granule cells per Purkinje's cell. The Purkinje's cells and the deep nuclear cells fire continuously at 50 to 100/sec.

   4. **Basket and stellate cells** (inhibitory)—lie along the parallel fibers and are stimulated by them to inhibit the adjacent Purkinje's cells.

   5. **Golgi's type II cells** (inhibitory)—in the granular layer and inhibit the granule cells and decrease the duration of an excitatory response.

H. The cerebellum stimulates the agonists while inhibiting the antagonists and then does the reverse.

I. There is probably cerebellar learning mediated by the climbing fibers adjusting the sensitivity of the Purkinje's cells. They fire at a rate of 1/s with strong excitatory impulses, and a rate change alters the long-term sensitivity of the Purkinje's cells to the mossy fibers. Once a task is mastered, climbing fibers no longer send error impulses. **The inferior olive receives input from the corticospinal tract and the motor centers of intent to compare the impulses.** If they correlate well, the inferior olive does not change its firing rate, but if the act needs to be altered, it may increase or decrease its rate.

J. Cerebellar **flocculonodular lobe**—important with rapid changes in body position as detected by the **vestibular apparatus**. It calculates the velocity and direction of movement to determine where the body will be to maintain equilibrium.

K. **Intermediate zone—compares the intentions of the cortex and red nucleus (by way of the efferent copy from the alpha motor neurons through the ventral spinocerebellar tract) with the actual performance as detected by the peripheral nervous system.** It sends corrections to the thalamic relay to the cortex, and to the red nucleus. It also has a damping function that prevents overshoot by anticipating momentum. Damage here causes intention tremor by allowing an overshoot in each direction. It also controls ballistic movements, short and fast actions where there is no time for feedback. These are all preplanned (i.e., eye saccades and finger typing). Damage here causes slow movements without the cerebellar agonist boost, decreased force, and slowness in stopping an action.

L. **Lateral zone**—has no input from the peripheral receptors or the primary motor cortex but **only from the premotor and association areas**. It is involved with the planning and time sequencing of movements. Damage here causes dyscoordination of speech and limbs. Planning is done with a two-way connection between the premotor cortex, the basal ganglia, and the sensory cortex. The dentate nucleus contains information about an action that will follow, not what is going on at the time. Damage will alter the timing control, making one unable to determine when a movement will end, and therefore preventing a smooth transition to the next movement. There is also extramotor function that predicts information from auditory and visual stimuli (i.e., how fast something is approaching).

M. In general, a lesion must involve at least one deep nucleus and the cortex to be symptomatic. There is no obvious change in function if one cortical hemisphere is removed. Deficits include dysmetria and ataxia (also seen with spinal cord tract lesions), dysdiadochokinesia (difficulty with rapid alternating movements), dysarthria (decreased coordination of breaths and words), intention tremor (by overshooting and lack of damping), nystagmus (failure of damping with tremor of the eyes, especially with flocculonodular damage), rebound (hitting oneself with a pulled and then released fist, occurs by the absence of the cerebellar component of the stretch reflex that fails to stop movement in an unwanted direction), and hypotonia (by loss of the ipsilateral dentate and interpositus nuclei's tonic discharge to the motor cortex and brain stem, it usually resolves within several months).

XIV. BASAL GANGLIA

A. Basal ganglia—control the intensity of the movement (scaling) and how fast it is performed (timing) (i.e., writing a big or little "a" and how quickly it is written). This timing and scaling is done by the caudate circuit with input from the association areas (i.e., the posterior parietal cortex provides the spatial relationship of the body to the surroundings). The basal ganglia have learned movements stored in them that must be relearned by the cortex if it is damaged.

B. **Putamen circuit**—executes motor activity patterns. Premotor cortex, supplementary motor cortex, and SS1 to the putamen to the GPi to the **VA and VL** thalamus to the primary motor, premotor, and supplementary motor cortices. There are also three smaller circuits: putamen to GPe to ST to thalamus to motor cortex; putamen to GPi to SN to thalamus to motor cortex; and GPe to ST to GPe.

C. Damage to the globus pallidus (GP) causes athetosis. Damage to the subthalamus (ST) causes hemiballismus. Damage to the caudate and putamen causes chorea. Damage to the substantia nigra (SN) causes rigidity and tremor.

D. **Caudate circuit**—involved with the cognitive control of motor patterns and integrates sensory information with memory to decide the motor activity. It chooses which muscle patterns will be used for each goal (i.e., if one sees a lion, one turns and climbs a tree). The caudate nucleus extends through all cortices (frontal, parietal, temporal, and occipital) and receives much input from the association areas. The prefrontal, premotor, and supplemental motor cortices and the parietal, temporal, and occipital association areas send fibers to the caudate and putamen and thence to the GPi to the VA and VL thalamus, to the prefrontal, premotor, supplemental motor cortices (but not to the primary motor cortex).

E. Neurotransmitters—SN sends dopaminergic fibers to the caudate and the putamen; the caudate and putamen send GABAergic fibers to the GP and SN; the caudate sends cholinergic fibers (ACh) to the putamen; the cortex sends cholinergic fibers to the caudate and putamen; the brain stem sends NE, serotonin (5-HT), and enkephalins to the basal ganglia. GABA and DA are inhibitory, whereas ACh is excitatory. All basal ganglia circuits to the cortex are inhibitory.

F. **Parkinson's disease (Fig. P–4)**—caused by degeneration of the **pars compacta** of the SN with decreased **DA** to the caudate and putamen. It is characterized by rigidity, tremor (3 to 6 cycles/s), akinesia, and postural instability. Because there is less DA to inhibit the caudate and putamen, there is more GABA to inhibit the GP and decrease the basal ganglia output. This allows more unopposed corticospinal stimulation with increased rigidity and tremor from oscillating circuits. Akinesia is due to impaired excitation-inhibition of the basal ganglia by the decreased DA. Increased ACh causes increased GABA from the GP and worsens symptoms. This disease is treated by raising DA levels (L-DOPA) or decreasing function of the VL and VA thalamus to inhibit the feedback loops. This last treatment is best for controlling tremors. Other targets include the GPi and the ST. See Chapter 4 for more information.

G. **Huntington's chorea**—caused by the loss of **GABAnergic neurons** in the caudate and putamen that produces less inhibition of the GP and the SN. The associated dementia may be due to ACh changes in the cortex.

XV. NEUROTRANSMITTER CHANGES IN DISEASE

A. Parkinson's disease—DA is decreased.

B. Huntington's disease and dementia—ACh is decreased.

C. Depression—decreased NE or serotonin (5-HT) or both in the raphe nucleus and locus ceruleus that go to the limbic system and cortex to stimulate pleasure and well-being centers. Treatment is with MAO inhibitors to decrease the destruction of NE and 5-HT, tricyclics to block the reuptake of 5-HT and

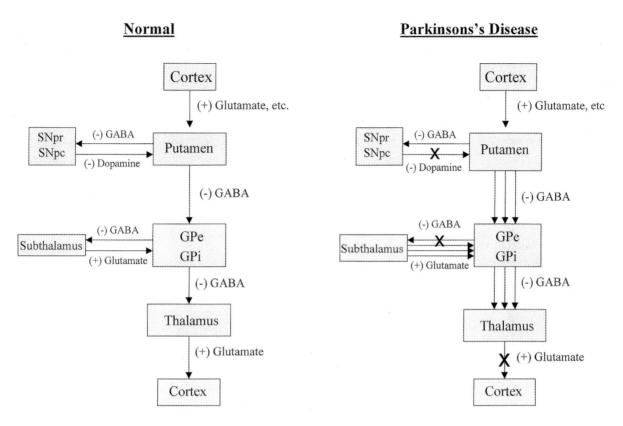

Figure P–4   Neurotransmitters in Parkinson's disease.

NE, or shock therapy to increase the NE transmission that occurs after seizures. Manic depression is treated with lithium to decrease the formation and action of NE and 5-HT.

D. Schizophrenia—increased DA and is characterized by auditory hallucinations, delusions of grandeur, paranoia, fear, etc. There is overactivity of the ventral tegmentum of the midbrain medial and superior to the SN (mesolimbic dopaminergic system) that stimulates mainly the medial and anterior limbic areas.

E. Alzheimer's disease—decreased ACh. There is a 75% loss of neurons in the nucleus basalis of Meynert beneath the GP in the substantia innominata that has input from the limbic system and output to the neocortex. ACh activates the neuronal mechanism for storage and recall of memories. There is also a decrease in somatostatin and substance P.

XVI. MOTOR CONTROL

A. Spinal cord—contains local patterns of muscle movement that are stimulated or inhibited by higher centers. Stored movements include reflexes, walking, etc.

B. Brain stem—maintains the axial tone for standing and equilibrium that is modified by vestibular input.

C. Corticospinal tract—issues commands and changes the intensity or timing of movements. It can bypass the spinal cord patterns by inhibition and can learn (unlike the spinal cord).

D. Cerebellum—modifies stretch reflexes to allow a movement to be load dependent, and it smoothes the equilibrium movements. It provides accessory motor commands to enable the intention to correlate with the exact target (a learned behavior). It also programs the next movement, especially with fast movements.

E. Basal ganglia—help the cortex to execute learned movements and are involved with the planning of parallel and sequential patterns of movement, modifying timing/rate and intensity/size, and planning appropriate actions. They require parietal lobe input because loss of either lobe causes contralateral neglect.

XVII. CORTICAL FUNCTIONS (FIG. P–5)

A. The cortex—2 to 5 mm thick and contains 100 billion neurons.

B. Three cell types—granular cells (stellate) have short axons, are intracortical, use glutamate (+) and GABA (−), and are more numerous in sensory and association areas where processing occurs. Fusiform cells are for output. Pyramidal cells are for output, are larger and more numerous, and send large axons to the spinal cord and subcortical association fibers.

C. The incoming cortical fibers arrive in layer 4. The output is from layer 5 (to the brain stem and spinal cord) and layer 6 (to the thalamus). Layers 1 to 3 provide intracortical association fibers to adjacent cortical areas.

D. The thalamus and cortex have reciprocal connections and function as a unit.

E. All sensory input goes to the thalamus except olfaction.

F. Association areas—distinct from the primary and secondary motor and sensory areas. They receive and analyze information from several different areas of cortex and various subcortical structures.

G. **Parieto-occipito-temporal association cortex**—between the somatosensory, visual, and auditory cortices. It determines the spatial coordinates of the body and its surroundings. If it is damaged, there is neglect of the opposite side of the body and its surroundings.

   1. Wernicke's area (Brodmann's area 22)—the language comprehension area and is located behind the primary auditory cortex in the posterior superior temporal lobe. It is the most important area for higher intellectual function because this is language based. It is in the left hemisphere in almost all right-handed people. Stimulation elicits complex thought, memory, visual scenes, and auditory hallucinations.

   2. **Angular gyrus** (visual association area)—posterior to Wernicke's area and anterior to the occipital lobe. It is in the posterior inferior parietal lobe and is used for the visual processing of words and supplies this information to Wernicke's area. Damage to this area causes dyslexia (inability to read) without a deficit in understanding spoken language. Damage to the auditory association area produces word deafness. The ability to name a word is located in the lateral temporal occipital junction.

Figure P–5   Functional Cortical Areas.

H. Language function—uses many different areas: Wernicke's area for thought formation and word choosing; Broca's area for vocalizing; the motor cortex, cerebellum, basal ganglia, and sensory system to control the pharyngeal and laryngeal movements.

I. **Prefrontal association area**—works with the motor cortex to plan complex patterns and sequences. It receives input from the parietal, temporal, and occipital association areas. Output is to the caudate loop for sequential and parallel movement complexes. It is also involved with thought elaboration.

　1. Broca's area—controls word formation and execution and coordinates the simultaneous stimulation of respiratory, pharyngeal, and laryngeal muscles. Part of it is in the prefrontal cortex and part in the premotor cortex.

　2. After a prefrontal lobotomy, there is impaired complex problem solving, decreased ambition, decreased ability to do sequential tasks to reach a goal, decreased ability to do parallel tasks, decreased aggression (limbic), decreased social responsiveness (especially in regards to sex and excretion), mood changes, decreased purpose, and decreased attention span (because this cortex has input from all areas and normally decides the motor response).

　3. Prefrontal cortex—needed to keep track of multiple simultaneous information and to recall it as needed. It is used to prognosticate, plan, and delay action until all sensory input is considered. It is used to consider the consequences of actions and solve complicated problems.

J. Limbic association area—located in the anterior basal temporal lobe, the basal frontal lobe, and the cingulate gyrus. It is involved in behavior, motivation, and emotion.

K. There is hemispheric dominance for Wernicke's area, the angular gyrus, speech function, and motor function. The left side is dominant in 95%, there is dual dominance in 5%, and there is rare right-sided dominance. Dominance may switch sides if the cortex is injured when young (usually before 2 years of age) . The left hemisphere is larger at birth 50% of the time. Dominance may develop because one hemisphere gets larger and attracts more input. The brain focuses on one area at a time, so the other area becomes silent. Both sides are connected by the corpus callosum, so there is no conflicting activity.

L. A major portion of our sensory experience is stored as language equivalents; therefore the language center develops closer to the temporal lobe than the occipital lobe because children first learn language by hearing before reading.

M. Nondominant parietotemporal occipital cortex—used for music, nonverbal visual expression, spatial relationships, body language, and voice intonations.

N. **Prosoprognosia**—inability to recognize faces and caused by **bilateral damage to the medial basal occipitotemporal cortex** between the limbic cortex in the temporal lobe and the visual cortex in the occipital lobe.

O. Corpus callosum—connects the respective cortical areas in the two hemispheres except for the anterior temporal lobe and amygdala, which are connected by the anterior commissure. It connects Wernicke's language information with the control of the left hand and also with the left visual and somatic input. The temporal lobe connections of the anterior commissure allow similar bilateral emotional output.

XVIII. THOUGHTS AND MEMORY

A. A thought is characterized as a stimulation pattern of many different parts of the cortex in a definite sequence.

B. Consciousness—the stream of awareness of our thoughts and surroundings.

C. The limbic system, thalamus, and reticular formation determine the quality of pleasure and pain, and provides crude localization.

D. The cortex determines specific localization, shape, etc.

E. Pain is elicited by midbrain and hypothalamic stimulation but very little by cortical stimulation.

F. Memory results from the change in capability of synaptic transmission from one neuron to the next as a result of previous activity. It causes new pathways to form, and these are called **memory traces**. Once established, it can be activated by the mind to reproduce memories. Some memories may be stored in the spinal cord and brain stem (i.e., blink reflex). The brain ignores some information, or else its memory would be filled up within minutes. The inhibition of the memory of useless sensory information is called habituation. Pain and pleasure are stored by the facilitation of the synaptic pathways (memory sensitization). The determination of whether to save a memory is made by the basal limbic areas. Each area of the thalamus reverberates with specific cortical areas and may help store memories.

    1. **Immediate memory (recall)**—lasts up to several minutes, and only while one is thinking of the facts such as a 7 to 10 number sequence. It is maintained by the continued activity in a

temporary memory trace by means of reverberating neurons. Presynaptic facilitation or inhibition may be involved. Synaptic potentiation may occur because frequent impulses cause an accumulation of Ca^{++} that increases the neurotransmitter release.

2. **Short-term memory**—lasts several weeks and is caused by chemical or physical changes. The snail Aplysia studied by Kandel was used as a model. In 3 weeks, a noxious stimulus would stimulate the sensory terminal and cause the facilitator terminal to store the information, or else the impulse would die out gradually. The stimulation of the facilitator terminal at the same time as the sensory terminal causes serotonin to be released to the presynaptic terminal by the facilitator nerve ending. This increases the cAMP inside the presynaptic sensory terminal and causes increased protein kinase levels that block K^+ channels for minutes to weeks. A longer action potential causes increased Ca^{++} influx, increased neurotransmitter release, and facilitates transmission.

3. **Long-term memory**—lasts longer than 3 weeks and is caused by structural changes at the synapses that either increase or decrease conduction. There is increased area of the vesicle release site, so there can be more neurotransmitter released (this decreases with less stimulation). There can be an increase in the number of neurotransmitter vesicles in the presynaptic terminals and an increased number of terminals.

G. The number of synapses increases with age as a child grows but decreases in the blind, deaf, etc. The number of neurons is greatest near birth, and they gradually diminish in number if not used, although they flourish with rapid learning.

H. The conversion of a memory from immediate to short-term or long-term needs "consolidation": A chemical, physical, or structural change that occurs over 5 minutes to 1 hour. The brain stores memory better with frequent rehearsals, especially with less information and more repetition. Also, the memory is stored better if placed in categories with similarities and differences.

I. The hippocampus stores new memories and is an important output area for the reward/punishment area of the limbic system. The motivation from a happy or sad experience excites the brain to store the experience as a memory. The decision of what is to be remembered is made by the **hippocampus** and the **DM thalamus**. Removal of both hippocampi decreases the long-term memory storage (anterograde amnesia) for verbal and symbolic memories.

J. Damage to the amygdala impairs new memory formation.

K. The temporal lobe and Wernicke's area are needed for normal consolidation and analysis.

L. Retrograde amnesia—affects more severely the more recent memories because the older memories are rehearsed so much that they become stored in many different parts of the brain. A hippocampal lesion can cause both anterograde and retrograde amnesia. A thalamic lesion only causes retrograde amnesia because it is used to help search the storehouses of memory.

M. Reflexive learning—as distinct from declarative learning, such as hand skills, is not verbal or symbolic. It is not affected by temporal lobe damage. Learning is by repetitive physical activity, not by symbolic rehearsal in the mind.

XIX. RETICULAR ACTIVATING SYSTEM AND NEUROTRANSMITTERS (FIG. P–6)

A. Input from the reticular activating system keeps the brain "on." If it is turned off or the brain stem is cut above the fifth nerve, the patient falls into a coma. It is located in the **middle and lateral pons and midbrain**. It sends signals up but also down to the spinal cord to maintain tone in the antigravity muscles and to activate the spinal reflexes. The output is to all of the subcortical structures but especially to the thalamus for diffuse spread. Large cells send rapid short-lasting signals with ACh to the thalamus. Small cells send slow fibers to the **intralaminar nuclei** of the thalamus and the **reticular nuclei** over the thalamic surface that last longer and control the background excitability of the brain. There is increased output with increased sensation, especially with pain. There is positive feedback by the cortex to the reticular system when it is active.

B. Inhibitory reticular formation —in the lower brain stem at the medial ventral medulla. Its neurotransmitter is serotonin, and it can reduce the tonic signals that are sent from the pons to the spinal cord to stimulate the antigravity muscles. It needs cortical input to function.

C. Brain activity is also controlled by excitatory and inhibitory neurotransmitters that are directly released into the brain or at the synapses with a longer duration (from minutes to hours). Norepinephrine is excitatory, is released diffusely, and is distributed by neurons arising from the locus ceruleus. Serotonin is inhibitory, released in the midline, and comes from the raphe nucleus. DA can be either excitatory or inhibitory and is mainly contained in neurons in the basal ganglia and the SN. Acetylcholine is excitatory and is released from the **basal nucleus of Meynert** and the gigantocellular nucleus of the reticular formation.

D. **Locus ceruleus**—located bilaterally at the posterior pontine midbrain junction. It sends diffuse projections that are predominantly excitatory (**NE**), although a few areas are inhibitory by certain receptors.

E. SN—sends inhibitory fibers to the caudate and putamen that release DA. DA, however, is excitatory in the hypothalamus and limbic system.

F. **Raphe nucleus** in the lower pons and medulla—inhibits with **serotonin**, mostly to the thalamus for sleep and restful functions but also to the cortex for sleep and to the spinal cord to decrease pain.

G. Gigantocellular layer of the reticular activating system in the pons and midbrain—stimulates with ACh. The neurons branch to send one limb to the cortex and one to the reticulospinal tract.

H. Other neurotransmitters—GABA, enkephalin, angiotensin 2, endorphins, EPI, ACTH, glutamate, and others.

XX. LIMBIC SYSTEM WITH HYPOTHALAMUS AND HIPPOCAMPUS

A. Limbic (border) system—the hypothalamus, septal area, paraolfactory area, epithalamus, anterior thalamic nucleus, hippocampus, and amygdala.

B. Orbitofrontal cortex—sends fibers to the subcallosal gyrus to the cingulate gyrus to the parahippocampus and uncus.

C. **Medial forebrain bundle**—a bidirectional tract connecting the septal nuclei and orbitofrontal gyrus through the middle of the hypothalamus to the reticular formation. It also connects the reticular formation to the thalamus, hypothalamus, and cortex.

D. Hypothalamus—connected to the reticular formation of the midbrain, pons, and medulla, as well as the diencephalon and cortex (especially the anterior thalamic nucleus and limbic cortex). It also connects by means of the infundibulum to the pituitary. It controls vegetative and endocrine functions and behavior.

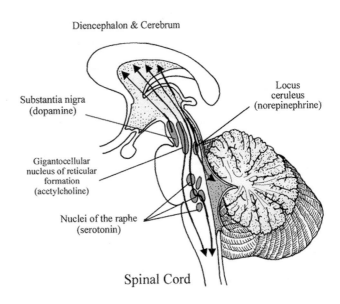

Figure P–6   Brain stem neurotransmitters.

E. Lateral hypothalamus—controls thirst, hunger, emotion, and sympathetic output.

F. Medial hypothalamus—controls satiety.

G. Stimulation of the anterior hypothalamus—causes a decrease in temperature, heart rate, and blood pressure, as well as distributing parasympathetic output.

H. Posterior hypothalamus—initiates an increase in temperature, heart rate, and blood pressure, as well as increases sympathetic tone.

I. Temperature—mainly controlled by the anterior hypothalamus, especially the preoptic area.

J. Body water concentration—a balance between the thirst impulses from the lateral hypothalamus and the renal excretion of water from the supraoptic nucleus that produces ADH.

K. Uterine contractility and milk ejection—controlled by the release of oxytocin from the paraventricular nucleus. Its production increases at the end of pregnancy, causing the uterus to contract and allowing the sucking reflex to deliver milk.

L. Feeding habits—dictated by the lateral hypothalamus that initiates searching behavior, the ventromedial hypothalamus that controls satiety, and the mamillary bodies that control feeding reflexes such as the licking of lips and swallowing.

M. Endocrine function—controlled by means of the portal blood that delivers hypothalamic releasing factors from the hypothalamic **arcuate nucleus** and **median eminence** of the infundibulum to the pituitary gland.

N. The limbic system determines whether a sensation is pleasant or unpleasant and thus controls our drives and motivations. The reward centers are located in the lateral and ventromedial hypothalamic nuclei and the medial forebrain bundle. Strong lateral nucleus stimulation causes rage and punishment (unpleasant feelings). Reward centers are also to a lesser degree located in the septum, amygdala, thalamus, basal ganglia, and midbrain. Punishment is located in the central gray and periventricular hypothalamus, as well as the amygdala and hippocampus. Punishment and fear can override pleasure and reward.

O. Tranquilizers (i.e., chlorpromazine)—inhibit both the reward and punishment centers and decrease motivation.

P. **Behavior**—controlled by the lateral hypothalamus (hunger, rage, and level of activity), the ventro-medial hypothalamus (satiety and peacefulness), the periventricular region and central gray midbrain (fear and punishment), and the anterior and posterior hypothalamic nuclei (sex drive).

Q. Rage—caused by stimulation of the lateral hypothalamic nuclei and the periventricular punishment areas and elicits defensive behavior, claw extension, tail lifting, hissing, spitting, growling, pupillary dilation, eye opening, piloerection, and attacking.

R. Fear and anxiety—elicited by stimulation of the midline preoptic nucleus and in animals cause a flight response. These impulses are counterbalanced by the ventromedial nucleus, amygdala, anterior cingulate gyrus, and anterior subcallosal gyrus.

S. Placidity and tameness—elicited by stimulation of the reward centers.

T. Learning—requires either reward or punishment stimulation to be remembered. Otherwise, the stimulus causes habituation and is ignored. If it elicits a reward feeling or punishment, stimulus repetition reinforces memory.

U. **Amygdala**—has bidirectional connections with the hypothalamus. It receives input from the olfactory tract to the corticomedial nucleus under the pyriform cortex. The basolateral nucleus is more important in humans and is not olfactory related. Input is from all the limbic cortex and the parietal, temporal, and occipital cortices (especially the visual and auditory association areas) that serve as the **limbic system's window to the outside world**. The output is to these same cortical areas, hippocampus, septal areas, thalamus, and hypothalamus.

V. Stimulation of the amygdala—may cause all of the hypothalamic effects (changes in blood pressure, heart rate, GI motility and secretion, defecation, micturition, pupillary changes, and anterior pituitary secretions), tonic movements (i.e., raising the head and bending the body), clonic movements, eating movements (licking, chewing, and swallowing), rage, pleasure, sexual feelings, ejaculation, ovulation, uterine contractions, and copulatory movements.

W. Bilateral amygdala ablation—causes **Klüver-Bucy syndrome**, characterized by a tendency to examine objects orally, decreased aggressiveness, tameness, diet change (they may become carnivorous), **psychic blindness** (loss of ability to determine what an object is used for by sight), **increased sex drive** (frequently inappropriate), curiosity, fearlessness, and forgetfulness.

X. Hippocampus—connects to the cortex and the limbic system (amygdala, hypothalamus, septum, and mamillary bodies). Incoming sensory information goes to the hippocampus and then to the anterior thalamus. Stimulation of various areas elicits many reactions similar to amygdaloid stimulation.

Y. The hippocampus has a low seizure threshold with long output signals. The seizures are psychomotor with olfactory (**uncinate fits**), visual, auditory, and tactile hallucinations. It may be more excitable because it is a three-layered paleocortex.

Z. The hippocampus functions as the critical decision maker early in life (whether to eat food, sexual impulses, detection of danger by smell with input from the olfactory areas) and later as the decider of what gets remembered. It senses reward/punishment and rehearses the immediate memories until they are stored. **Without the hippocampus, one is unable to consolidate short-term memories.**

AA. Bilateral removal impairs the ability to learn new verbal symbolism (anterograde amnesia), but one can still recall with immediate memory, although some retrograde amnesia may occur for events in the past year.

BB. Limbic cortex—an **association area** for the control of behavior and is the transitional zone from the cortex to the limbic system. Ablation of the temporal tip causes Klüver-Bucy syndrome, of the posterior orbitofrontal cortex causes insomnia and restlessness, and of the anterior cingulate and subcallosal gyri causes rage by the release of the septal nuclei and the hypothalamus. The anterior temporal cortex is mostly used for olfactory and gustatory associations. The parahippocampal gyri are for auditory associations and complex thought (with Wernicke's area). The middle and posterior cingulate gyri are for sensorimotor associations.

XXI. BRAIN ACTIVITY STATES

A. Sleep

1. Sleep—when one is unconscious but arousable by stimuli. An alternation exists between slow-wave sleep and REM sleep throughout the night.

2. **Slow-wave sleep**—makes up 75% of sleep, is deep and restful, occurs for the first hour, and is characterized by decreased blood pressure, respiratory rate, and BMR. Dreams occur in this sleep, but they are not remembered.

3. **REM sleep**—makes up 25% of sleep, occurs every 90 minutes, lasts 5 to 30 minutes although shorter if one is more tired and longer toward end of night, has increased dreaming, is harder to awaken with sensory stimuli, and is characterized by decreased muscle tone, irregular respiratory rate and heart rate, and increased BMR (20%). The EEG is like the awake state (paradoxical sleep).

4. Stimulus for sleep—the old theory is passive, stating that sleep occurred when the ascending reticular activating system (ARAS) fatigued. The new theory involves active inhibition of the ARAS and is based on the fact that sleep never occurs if the midpons is severed and removed from cortical control.

5. Muramyl peptides and other sleep factors accumulate when one is awake, and they increase in the CSF and urine in sleep-deprived people.

6. Sleep cycle—may occur by gradual fatigue of the ARAS and the accumulation of sleep factors with awakening when there has been a decrease in the sleep factors and a reinvigoration of the ARAS.

Brain Waves during Wakefulness and Sleep

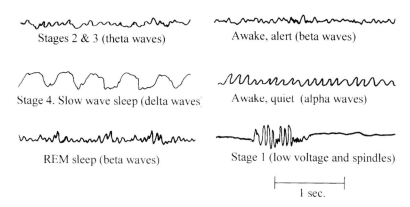

Stages 2 & 3 (theta waves)

Awake, alert (beta waves)

Stage 4. Slow wave sleep (delta waves)

Awake, quiet (alpha waves)

REM sleep (beta waves)

Stage 1 (low voltage and spindles)

1 sec.

7. Raphe nucleus in the midline lower pons and upper medulla—connected to the reticular formation, thalamus, cortex, hypothalamus, limbic system, and dorsal horns of the spinal cord (for pain modulation). The raphe nucleus uses serotonin as its neurotransmitter and stimulation elicits sleep.

8. Stimulation of the solitary tract nucleus, which receives input from visceral sensation by CN VII, IX, and X, increases sleep but not if the raphe nucleus is destroyed.

9. Other structures involved with sleep—the rostral hypothalamus (suprachiasmal portion) and the intralaminar thalamic nuclei.

10. Lesion of the locus ceruleus—decreases REM sleep because it activates certain cortical areas during REM sleep without causing wakefulness.

11. Sleep deprivation—causes psychosis, decreased thought, increased sympathetic output, decreased parasympathetic output but no physical harm to the body.

B. Brain waves/EEG (**Fig. P–7**)

1. Amplitude of brain waves—0 to 200 μV and the frequency is 0.3 to $>$50/s, usually without a pattern. The brain waves only form when many neurons fire synchronously and are mainly from layers 1 and 2. Increased activity causes increased wave frequency but decreased voltage because they are more asynchronous.

2. **Alpha waves**—have a frequency of 8 to 12/s and an amplitude of 50 μV. They occur when one is awake and quiet, mostly in the **occipital** lobes. **They are suppressed with eye opening or thought and disappear with sleep.** They are changed to asynchronous beta waves when attention moves elsewhere (increased frequency and decreased voltage). They will not form without a corticothalamic connection because they are elicited by the spontaneous firing of nonspecific thalamic nuclei.

3. **Beta waves**—frequency of 12 to 25/s but have decreased amplitude. They occur in the **frontal** and parietal areas when one is **active**.

4. **Theta waves**—frequency of 4 to 7/s, increased amplitude, and occur in the **parietal and temporal** areas in children. They may occur with stress in adults and are increased with brain disorders.

5. **Delta waves**—frequency of 1 to 3/s and have increased amplitude. They occur with **deep sleep**, infancy, **brain disease**, and subcortical transections separating the cortex from the thalamus (deep sleep may separate the cortex from underlying control).

6. **Slow-wave sleep**—four stages: stage 1 sleep is very light sleep with elimination of α waves; stage 2 sleep is characterized by **sleep spindles** (short alpha bursts) and **K complexes**; stage 3 and 4 sleep are characterized by slow-wave high-amplitude **delta waves**. Stages 2 and 3 may have theta waves.

7. REM sleep—beta waves that are desynchronized like in the awake state.

C. Epilepsy

1. Seizure—sudden synchronous alteration of brain electrical activity from increased activity of part or all of the CNS.

2. **Generalized tonic/clonic (grand mal) seizures**—involve the entire brain. They are at first tonic then tonic/clonic with high-voltage synchronized discharges of 100 μV with increased frequency. They may occur by activation of the reticular formation or the thalamus. The overall prevalence of epilepsy is about 1 to 2% of the population. Seizure frequency is increased with emotion, alkalosis, drugs, fever, loud noise, light flashes, and trauma. They are caused by reverberating circuits and end by fatigue or active inhibition.

3. **Absence (petite mal) seizures**—3 to 30 seconds of unconsciousness followed by blinking and head twitching. They are activated by the basal forebrain and are more common in late childhood to 30 years of age. There is a typical **3/s spike and dome waveform on the EEG**. They rarely initiate a generalized tonic/clonic seizure.

4. **Focal seizures**—caused by either congenital circuit derangements, a variety of brain injuries that cause gliosis and neuronal damage, tumors, infection, trauma with contusion, or strokes. They are due to local reverberating circuits and may spread from the upper limbs to the mouth and lower limbs (Jacksonian epilepsy). They may lead to midbrain excitement, which elicits a grand mal seizure. Psychomotor seizures are characterized by amnesia, rage, anxiety, and incoherent speech.

5. See Chapter 6 for more on seizures.

XXII. AUTONOMIC NERVOUS SYSTEM

A. **Sympathetic nervous system**—originates in the hypothalamus, which sends fibers down to the ipsilateral **intermediolateral cell column** that extends from **T1 to L2**. The neurons in this cell column send fibers in the anterior root to the spinal nerves to the **preganglionic fibers (white ramus)** to the paravertebral chain of ganglia (fibers may bypass the paravertebral ganglia and synapse in other ganglia or in the prevertebral ganglia) such as the celiac and hypogastric plexi to the **postganglionic fibers (gray ramus)** back to the spinal nerves.

B. **C fibers**—travel in the skeletal nerves to control blood pressure, sweating, and piloerection. Eight percent of fibers in the skeletal nerves are sympathetic.

C. **Splanchnic nerves**—preganglionic fibers that pass through the sympathetic chain without synapsing to the adrenal medullae, where they act on postganglionic cells that release mainly EPI and some NE.

D. The sympathetic system does not have as many segments as the spinal nerves. Its distribution is determined by where an organ was in the embryo, such as the heart in the neck and the abdominal contents in the lower thorax. Various levels are T1, head; T2, neck; T3-6, thorax; T7-11, abdomen; and T12-L2, lower extremities. There is sympathetic innervation to the entire body. The sympathetic nerves only travel with blood vessels in the head and neck.

E. **Parasympathetic system**—75% **cranial** (CN III, VII, IX, and X) and 25% **sacral** (S2 to 4). Unlike the sympathetic system, the parasympathetic system **only innervates part of the body**. Parasympathetic innervation is to the head, neck, and viscera but **not to the limbs**. The oculomotor nerve (CN III) supplies the pupillary sphincter and the ciliary muscle. The facial nerve (CN VII) innervates the lacrimal, nasal, submandibular, and sublingual glands. The glossopharyngeal nerve (CN IX) innervates the parotid gland. The vagus nerve (CN X) provides parasympathetic innervation of the body down to the midcolon. The sacral roots go to the **nervi erigentes** (pelvic nerves) that leave the sacral plexus to supply the descending colon, bladder, lower uterus, and external genitalia.

F. The sacral preganglionic fibers go to the organs that they innervate and synapse in their walls. They have short 1-mm to several centimeter postganglionic fibers that are in the substance of the organ. The synapses for CN parasympathetics are in the ganglia. No parasympathetic fibers pass through the ganglia without synapsing.

G. Parasympathetic stimulation—elicits copious secretions in the mouth and stomach, but the intestines are controlled mainly by local factors.

H. **Sweat**—mainly controlled by the **sympathetic system** (with **ACh** as the postganglionic neurotransmitter in this rare case) except for the parasympathetic innervation to the palms of the hands. The thick apocrine secretions are by sympathetic impulses only.

I. Autonomic system's neurotransmitters—all preganglionic fibers use ACh; postganglionic parasympathetic fibers use ACh; most postganglionic sympathetic fibers use NE, except for sweat, piloerectors, blood vessels that use ACh acting on muscarinic receptors.

J. **ACh**—made in the terminal nerve endings outside the vesicles via acetyl-CoA + choline by choline acetyltransferase (made in the soma) to ACh. It is broken down by acetylcholinesterase (in the glycosaminoglycans of the connective tissue) to choline + acetate.

K. **NE** synthesis—started in the axoplasm of the terminal endings (tyrosine to DOPA to DA) and is finished in the vesicles (DA to NE to EPI). Its removal is by (1) presynaptic reuptake (50 to 80%),

(2) diffusion into blood (20 to 50%), and (3) destruction by mono-amine oxidase (MAO) (minimal). It is rapidly cleared and lasts 10 to 30 s in the blood before catechol O-methyltransferase destroys it in the liver.

L. The receptor protein penetrates the cell membrane and a shape change after binding causes an increased ion permeability or enzyme activation. EPI causes an increase in cAMP that may increase or decrease different reactions. The reaction in each organ depends on the receptor protein.

M. Acetylcholine receptors

   1. **Nicotinic receptors**—nicotine stimulates these. They are located in the NMJ and preganglionic endings both sympathetic and parasympathetic fibers. There autonomic receptor has five subunits $\alpha_2\beta\gamma\delta$. The α-subunit is the binding site for ACh (thus each receptor can bind two ACh molecules) and is composed of four hydrophobic transmembrane proteins. The receptor is blocked by hexamethonium (depolarizing, not reversible with anticholinesterase).

   2. **Muscarinic receptors**—muscarine stimulates these. They are located in all the postganglionic parasympathetic endings and the postganglionic sympathetic endings to sweat glands, piloerectors, and blood vessels. The receptor's effect is mediated by a G protein with a secondary messenger system. Activation of one G protein will inhibit all other G proteins in the cell. This receptor is blocked by pertussis toxin.

N. **Adrenergic receptors**—NE stimulates alpha $>$ beta; EPI stimulates alpha and beta equally.

O. Adrenal medulla—releases 80% EPI and 20% NE. Its effects last 5 to 10 times longer than other sympathetic stimulation because its products are cleared slowly, and this produces more systemic effects including increased BMR. Both the hormonal and the direct stimulation of the sympathetic system work together.

P. The autonomic system works with a low stimulation rate of 10 to 20/s as opposed to the 50 to 500 impulses/s needed for muscle stimulation. It is always active with a basal rate of sympathetic and parasympathetic tone, and this allows one system to increase or decrease for control. There is also a basal secretion rate of EPI and NE from the adrenal gland. After the sympathetic and parasympathetic input is cut from an organ, it gradually compensates with intrinsic tone to a level near baseline. The organ also develops denervation supersensitivity with increased responses to NE, EPI, and ACh.

Q. Autonomic reflexes

   1. Baroreceptor reflex—specific organs sense stretch in the aorta, carotid, etc., in the face of increased BP; stretch elicits a decrease in sympathetic tone to lower the BP.

   2. GI reflexes—the smell of food or its presence in the mouth stimulates the vagal, glossopharyngeal, and salivatory nuclei to increase oral and gastric secretions. Feces in the rectum causing distention elicits an impulse to the spinal cord to the parasympathetic system to increase peristalsis to empty the bowel. Accumulation of urine in the bladder elicits a similar response.

   3. Mass response (sympathetic)—stress can cause increased BP, increased blood flow to the muscle, decreased blood flow to the GI tract and kidney, increased BMR, increased serum glucose and glycolysis, increased muscle strength and mental activity, and increased blood coagulation.

4. Focal response (sympathetic)—change in body temperature alters sweating and skin blood flow. Some reflexes do not involve the spinal cord but may only go to the ganglia.

5. Parasympathetic responses—usually more specific.

R. Drugs that affect the autonomic system

1. Sympathomimetics—act on the adrenergic receptors. Phenylephrine stimulates alpha receptors. Isoproterenol stimulates beta 1 and 2. Albuterol stimulates beta 2. Increased NE release is caused by ephedrine, tyramine, and amphetamine.

2. Reserpine—blocks the synthesis and storage of NE and causes release from the vesicles.

3. Guanethidine—decreases NE release.

4. Alpha blockers—phenoxybenzamine and phentolamine.

5. Beta 1 and 2 blockers—propranolol.

6. Beta 1 blockers only—metoprolol.

7. Sympathetic and parasympathetic ganglionic blockers—hexamethonium, TEA ion, and pentolinium. These are more effective on the sympathetic system so they cause a decrease in BP.

8. Muscarinic receptor agonists (parasympathetic)—pilocarpine and methacholine. These also cause sweating by sympathetic organs and vasodilation.

9. Muscarinic ACh receptor blockers—atropine and scopolamine.

10. Anticholinesterases (reversible)—neostigmine, pyridostigmine, and physostigmine.

11. Anticholinesterase (irreversible)—organophosphates.

12. Nicotinic ACh receptor agonists—ACh, nicotine, and methacholine.

13. Nicotinic ACh ganglionic receptor blocker—hexamethonium; depolarizing and not reversed by anticholinesterase.

14. Depolarizing nicotinic ACh receptor blockers—succinylcholine and decamethonium, nonreversible with anticholinesterase. Their action is amplified with decreased muscle temperature.

15. Nondepolarizing nicotinic ACh receptor blocker—α-Bungarotoxin (curare), competitive inhibition.

16. Botulism toxin—decreased ACh release from the presynaptic terminal, also with aminoglycosides and Eaton-Lambert syndrome.

17. Cholera toxin—decreased GTP hydrolysis.

18. Tetanus toxin—blocks exocytosis by preventing fusion of the vesicle with the cell membrane.

19. Diphtheria toxin—inactivates tRNA transferase.

20. Strychnine—glycine antagonist, increases muscle rigidity.

21. Cocaine—blocks DA uptake as an α_1-uptake inhibitor.

22. TEA—blocks voltage-gated K^+ channels.

23. Tetrodotoxin—blocks voltage-gated Na^+ channels.

24. Cyanide—blocks the Na/K pump and impairs active transport.

XXIII. CEREBRAL BLOOD FLOW (CBF)

A. Cessation of blood flow to the brain of 5 to 10/s causes unconsciousness. The neurons need O_2.

B. **CBF**—normally **50 to 55 mL/100 g/min**. Neural function is impaired if CBF is $<$ **23 mL/100 g/min**. Irreversible damage occurs at CBF $<$ **8 mL/100 g/min** where the ionic pump fails.

C. **Ischemic penumbra**—the zone of neurons receiving between 8 and 23 mL/100 g/min of flow and where there is **isoelectric silence**. The cells here can still have function salvaged with the return of blood flow. This also depends on duration of ischemia, temperature, glucose concentration, location, and other factors.

D. CBF—normally is 15% of the cardiac output (CO), and the brain consumes 20% of the O_2 used by the body.

E. **CBF—increased by elevated $paCO_2$ or serum H^+ and lowered by decreased paO_2.**

F. $CO_2 + H_2O \rightarrow H_2CO_3$ (carbonic acid) $\rightarrow H^+ + HCO_3^-$. H^+ causes vasodilation. Any acid increases the CBF (lactic, etc). Acid decreases neural activity so it is fortunate that it increases CBF.

G. Oxygen use—normally 3.5 cc O_2/100 g/min.

H. CBF is **autoregulated** (remains constant) at mean arterial pressures of 60 to 140 mm Hg assuming a normal ICP.

I. Sympathetic fibers—innervate the brain's blood vessels but usually have little effect because local autoregulation keeps the CBF in normal range. However, increased blood pressure with exercise or other causes forces the sympathetic system to act to decrease the CBF in the face of the higher systemic pressure.

J. CBF and $CMRO_2$—highest in the gray matter, four times that of the white matter. The posterior pituitary gland receives the highest blood flow.

K. The brain mass is 2% of the body mass but accounts for 15% of its total metabolism. **No anaerobic glycolysis occurs in neurons**, and only low stores of glycogen and O_2 are present. Therefore, neurons require a constant supply of O_2 and glucose. All cells except neurons need insulin to uptake glucose. Glucose crosses the BBB by facilitated transport.

XXIV. SKELETAL MUSCLE (FIG. P–8)

A. Each muscle fiber is innervated by one nerve ending that synapses near the longitudinal midpoint of the fiber.

B. One myofibril has 1500 myosin and 3000 actin filaments.

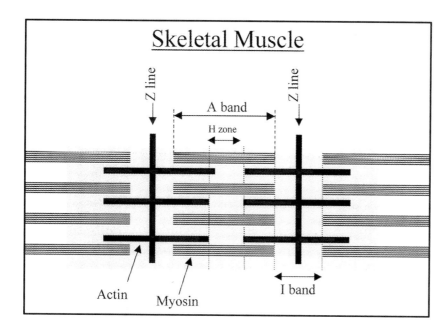

Figure P–8   Skeletal muscle.

C. **Light bands**—contain only actin. **Dark bands** have both myosin and actin. **I bands** have only actin and are isotropic to polarized light. **A bands** have actin and myosin and are anisotropic to polarized light. **H bands** have just myosin.

D. Sarcomere—muscle unit that lies between two **Z discs**.

E. Myofibrils of actin and myosin are in the sarcoplasm of the muscle fiber.

F. **Sacroplasmic reticulum (SR)**—the extensive endoplasmic reticulum in muscle (skeletal, cardiac, or smooth muscle).

G. **Myosin molecule**—has two heads, and there are 200 molecules per myosin filament. The myosin head has ATPase activity.

H. **Actin filament**—contains actin, **tropomyosin**, and **troponin C** (which binds four Ca^{++} ions).

I. **Sliding filament mechanism**—the accepted model for all muscle contraction.

　　1. The ACh receptor opens Na^+ channels and causes an action potential. This depolarizes the cell and adjacent SR at the muscle triads.

　　2. The sarcoplasmic reticulum releases Ca^{++} that binds troponin and moves the tropomyosin off of actin's binding site for myosin.

　　3. The myosin heads bind the actin and pull it along in a ratchet-like fashion. ATP cleavage on the myosin head causes it to become cocked before binding the actin. When the myosin binds the actin, a power stroke pulls the tilted myosin head, releasing ADP and Pi and causing the actin and myosin to slide along each other.

　　4. Then the ATP binds the myosin head and is cleaved, causing the myosin head to release the actin and to re-cock. Both the attachment and detachment of myosin to actin require ATP.

　　5. After contraction, there is active pumping of the Ca^{++} back to the SR, where it is stored with calsequestrin so very little is left in the cytosol. The Ca^{++} pulse and the contraction last 1/20 second.

J. Maximum contraction—occurs with maximum actin/myosin overlap of 2.2 to 2.0 μm. The normal resting muscle length, which is around the midpoint of the muscle length spectrum, has the highest force of contraction. The velocity of contraction decreases with increased load.

K. Muscle contraction occurs when the muscle membrane becomes depolarized and the current spreads inside to the SR, which releases Ca^{++}. The RMP is -80 to -90 mV (the same as large myelinated nerve fibers). The duration of the action potential is 1 to 5 ms (five times as long as in myelinated fibers). The velocity of the impulse is 3 to 5 m/s (1/18th that of nerve speed). The current spreads inside the muscle cell to all the fibrils by means of the **transverse tubules** (T tubules) that are extensions of the cell membrane filled with extracellular fluid and attached to the SR.

L. Muscle needs energy for myosin's ATP, the Ca^{++} SR pump, and the cell membrane RMP Na/K pump. Phosphocreatine and ATP stores last 8 seconds. Glycogenolysis is depleted at 60 seconds. Oxidative metabolism supplies energy over more prolonged times by use of carbohydrates and proteins for the short term and fats for the long term.

M. Only 25% of the energy created is used to do work; 75% is released as heat.

N. Isometric contractions—have no muscle length change. Isotonic contractions have no muscle tension change.

O. Duration of contraction of the ocular muscle—1/40 second, whereas that of the soleus is 1/5 second.

P. **Motor unit**—one alpha motor neuron and numerous muscle fibers (from 1600 in the quadriceps to six or so in the extraocular muscles where fine control is needed). Current spread occurs with other units so they help each other out and do not act separately.

Q. Multiple fiber summation—occurs because the smaller and weaker motor units are more excitable so they are stimulated first. This allows a gradation of force development. Units contract asynchronously so movement is smooth.

R. Frequency summation can occur and overlap can cause tetany.

S. Muscle fibers hypertrophy by increasing the number of intracellular fibrils not the number of cells (true hyperplasia does not occur).

T. Denervation—causes atrophy and replacement by fat and fibrous tissue. Re-innervation no longer helps after 1 to 2 years. Fibrous replacement may shorten the muscle fibers, causing contractures; therefore one must be sure to keep the muscle stretched during the atrophy process. An example is the frozen shoulder after a brachial plexus injury. After poliomyelitis, axons will sprout to cover other muscle units and form macromotor units with decreased fine control.

U. Skeletal muscle—innervated by large myelinated nerves. The **motor end plate** is insulated from the extracellular fluid by Schwann cells. The synaptic cleft is 20 to 30 nm wide. There are 300,000 ACh-containing vesicles at the axon terminal per motor end plate. Each action potential releases 300 vesicles into the synaptic cleft. Each vesicle contains **1 quantum = 10,000 ACh molecules**. The action potential in the axon terminal causes an increased Ca^{++} conductance by means of the voltage-gated Ca^{++} channels. This causes the ACh vesicles to fuse to the membrane near the dense bars for exocytosis.

V. Vesicles—formed in the neuronal cell body by the Golgi apparatus and transported to the axon terminal by axonal transport. ACh is synthesized in the cytosol and actively transported into the vesicles where they are concentrated 10,000 molecules (1 quantum) per vesicle. Occasionally, a vesicle fuses spontaneously with the membrane surface, causing an MEPP. A full end plate potential surpasses the threshold for muscle depolarization and causes an AP in the muscle fiber.

W. After the axon depolarizes and releases ACh to the NMJ causing muscle depolarization, the ACh is destroyed by acetylcholinesterase in the basal lamina filling the synaptic cleft and also is cleared by diffusion. The choline is reabsorbed by the axon terminal for reuse. The entire sequence occurs in 5 to 10 ms. The membrane of the vesicle is retrieved from the cell membrane by endocytosis as the coated pits with cathrin protein contract.

X. The muscle membrane has **subneural clefts** to increase its surface area. The ACh receptors are near the subneural clefts. They form a tubular channel through the cell membrane. ACh binding opens a tunnel through the channel. Na^+, K^+, and Ca^{++} can move through but not Cl^- because a negative charge is present in the mouth of the channel. Only Na^+ moves in, however, causing an end plate potential. If depolarization is large enough, an AP develops. The α-subunit is the ACh binding site so there are **two binding sites per ACh receptor**. There are four hydrophobic transmembrane proteins. The transmembrane part of the receptor protein is the most conserved. The cytoplasmic loop is the least conserved. The N and C terminals are extracellular.

Y. **Curare**—blocks the ACh receptor. **Botulism toxin** decreases ACh release. Both of these cause paralysis. **Neostygmine** blocks acetylcholinesterase for several hours. **Fluorophosphate** irreversibly blocks acetylcholinesterase for weeks and is treated with **PAM**.

Z. Myasthenia gravis (MG)—caused by antibodies to the ACh receptor. Treatment is with an acetylcholinesterase inhibitor such as neostigmine.

XXV. SMOOTH MUSCLE

A. Smooth muscle cells—smaller than skeletal muscle fibers.

B. Multi-unit smooth muscle—multiple, independent fibers innervated by a single nerve ending. The individual smooth muscle cells are connected by gap junctions (electrical synapses) that allow synchronous contraction of cells. No APs or spontaneous contractions are present. This group of smooth muscle includes the ciliary muscle, iris, and piloerectors.

C. Single-unit smooth muscle—syncytial, with a mass of fibers that contract together. The cell membranes are adherent and there are gap junctions for ion flow between cells. They may depolarize with or without an AP and thus may develop spontaneous contractions. This group includes the walls of the gut, uterus, and blood vessels.

D. Smooth muscle cells have no troponin. These cells have 15 times more actin than myosin. The dense body acts as a Z disc to anchor the actin. They have slower and longer contractions, slower cycling of cross-bridges (by decreased ATPase), increased time the cross-bridges are attached (increased force), less energy required, slower onset of contractions and relaxation, and can shorten much more than skeletal muscle with generation of full force. Skeletal muscle only contracts usefully over $\frac{1}{3}$ of its length. Smooth muscle can contract $\frac{2}{3}$ of its length because it has interspersed units that are not at the same point and longer actin filaments.

E. Contraction—regulated by Ca^{++} (although there is no troponin) after nerve stimulation, hormones, stretching, and chemical changes. Each calmodulin molecule reacts with four Ca^{++} ions. Ca^{++} binds the calmodulin and the complex joins and activates myosin kinase to phosphorylate the myosin heads and create a cycle. Then the Ca^{++} ion concentration decreases, all reverses, and the myosin phosphatase cleaves the phosphorus to relax. The time to relax is proportional to the myosin phophatase concentration.

F. Smooth muscle neuromuscular junction (NMJ)—formed by autonomic nerves that branch to form diffuse junctions that secrete neurotransmitters into the interstitial fluid a few nanometers away. These diffuse to the outer cell and either diffuse inside to the inner cell or cause an AP. No branching end feet are present as in skeletal muscle nerves, but instead varicosities are present. Some lie on the membrane of the muscle and form contact junctions that have quicker transmission.

G. ACh and NE—may be either stimulatory or inhibitory by different membrane receptors that control the ion channels.

H. RMP is -50 to -60 mV. APs occur only in the single-unit type (visceral smooth muscle). The action potential is mainly by increased Ca^{++} conductance because there are few voltage-gated Na^+ channels. They open more slowly than Na^+ channels so the AP is slower.

I. The slow wave potentials from the decreased pumping out of Na^+ ions may cause a spontaneous AP at -35 mV, allowing the cell to act as a pacemaker.

J. Excitation may occur with stretching that may decrease the intracellular negative charge.

K. Multiunit smooth muscle depolarizes without an AP in response to a nerve stimulus because it is too small a fiber to generate a sustaining action potential.

L. Most smooth muscle contraction is not by APs or neural input but by local tissue factors. These include decreased O_2, increased CO_2, increased H^+, adenosine, lactate, or K^+, decreased Ca^{++}, and temperature. All these factors cause dilation. Also hormones such as NE, EPI, ACh, 5-HT, histamine, angiotensin, and ADH may affect smooth muscle if a chemically gated receptor is present.

M. Ca^{++} for skeletal muscle contraction comes from the SR, but for smooth muscle contraction it comes from the extracellular space and is limited by the conductance speed through the Ca^{++} channels, so it is slower and has a latent period 50 times that of skeletal muscle. Smooth muscle has a rudimentary SR. Serum Ca^{++} concentration has no effect on skeletal muscle, but if is low, it causes decreased smooth muscle contraction. The slow pumps to clear the Ca^{++} cause a longer contraction.

XXVI. CARDIAC MUSCLE

A. Cardiac muscle—striated muscle, with cells separated by intercalated discs with minimal resistance to electricity that passes through gap junctions with ion flow. The syncytium permits easy flow of current.

B. Atrial syncytium—separated from the ventricular syncytium by a fibrous bundle around the valves, so the only pathway for current is by way of the AV node and conducting system.

C. The RMP in cardiac cells is -85 to -95 mV compared with the -90 to -100 mV in Purkinje's cells.

D. The AP with its plateau lasts longer than in skeletal muscle because of increased conductance through **slow Ca^{++}** and Na$^+$ channels and fast Na$^+$ channels and decreased conductance of K$^+$ initially. It has a slower velocity than in skeletal muscle. The atria have less refractory time than the ventricles so they can beat faster. The duration of the AP and contraction is 0.2 second in the atria and 0.3 second in the ventricle.

E. Excitation-contraction coupling—occurs with T tubules that help spread the AP to the myofibrils and with the longitudinal SR tubules with Ca^{++} release. Unlike skeletal muscle, there is also a Ca^{++} influx from outside the cell. There are less SR Ca^{++} stores but more T-tubules. Cardiac muscle depends more on extracellular Ca^{++}. T-tubules have mucopolysaccharides with negative charges to attract Ca^{++}.

F. Sino-atrial (SA) node—in the superior lateral right atrium below and lateral to the SVC. It has no contractile elements. It has the fastest automatic rhythm, so it controls the heart rate. The RMP is -55 mV because of a natural leak to Na$^+$ and at -40 mV the Ca^{++} channels open. Repolarization is by opening of K$^+$ channels. Fast Na$^+$ channels are blocked at > -60 mV, so only slow Ca^{++} and Na$^+$ channels open. The SA node has a slow action potential and a slow recovery.

G. Current spreads from the sinus node more quickly through anterior, middle, and posterior internodal pathways to the AV node and more slowly along the atrial fibers to the AV node. The AV node is at the posterior septal wall of the right atrium. It delays the signal 0.13 second. The delay is caused by slow transmission from (1) small fiber size, (2) few gap junctions, and (3) low RMP so there is less force to drive ions in. The impulse then travels along the Purkinje's fibers in the right and left bundle branches that are very large fibers with rapid transmission and have increased gap junctions.

H. AV node—prevents re-entry and the fibrous barrier prevents ventriculoatrial spread. The AV node self-fires at 40 to 60/min, the Purkinje's cells self-fire at 15 to 40/min, and the sinus node self-fires at 70 to 80/min. The ventricular escape rhythm is 15 to 40 bpm and is due to the septal Purkinje's fibers taking over.

I. Adams-Stokes syndrome—intermittent sudden AV block with a 5-to 30-second delay before the Purkinje system initiates its own beat. Patients may faint or die.

J. Parasympathetic system—innervates the SA and AV nodes to block both by increasing the K$^+$ conductance, which causes hyperpolarization of the cell membrane.

K. Sympathetic system—innervates the entire heart, with NE that increases Na$^+$ and Ca^{++} conductance. It can increase the rate three times and the contractility two times.

XXVII. CIRCULATION

A. Circulatory system—has intrinsic control by local factors and extrinsic control by the nervous system. The parasympathetic input is only important for heart function. The sympathetic system innervates the entire circulatory system. The sympathetic chain sends sympathetic nerves to the viscera and spinal nerves to the periphery. The sympathetic system innervates all vessels except capillaries, precapillary sphincters, and met-arterioles. Small arteries respond by changing blood flow and large veins by changing blood volume. The normal sympathetic vasoconstrictor tone contributes 50% of the total vessel tone; therefore a sympathetic block can lower the BP 50%.

B. Vasomotor center—in the reticular formation of the medulla and caudal pons.

    1. Vasoconstrictor area (C-1)—in the anterolateral upper medulla and sends NE to the spinal cord.

    2. Vasodilator area (A-1)—in the anterolateral lower medulla and projects up to the vasoconstrictor area for inhibition.

    3. Sensory area (A-2)—in the tractus solitarius at the posterolateral pons and medulla with input from CN IX and X. Each area originates bilaterally.

C. Lateral vasomotor center—sends sympathetic input to the heart, whereas the medial vasomotor center (near dorsal X) sends parasympathetic input to the heart. The vasomotor center is affected by the reticular formation of the diencephalon, mesencephalon, and pons (superolateral excites and inferomedial inhibits). The hypothalamus and limbic system may either excite or inhibit this region.

D. Sympathetic outflow—(1) constricts almost all arterioles and increases the PVR, (2) constricts veins, (3) increases the heart rate and contractility, and (4) is the fastest way to increase BP.

E. **Baroreceptor reflex**—uses spray-type nerve endings in the walls of arteries, especially the carotid sinus above the CCA bifurcation and in the aortic arch. Stretching of the carotid sinus stimulates **Hering's nerve** (CN IX), which synapses in the solitary tract. There is progressively increased firing as the mean BP increases from 60 to 180 mm Hg. The aortic receptors stimulate the vagus nerve to the solitary tract to inhibit the vasocontrictor center and stimulate the vasodilatory center if the mean BP is 90 to 210 mm Hg (normal is 100 mm Hg). The firing rate increases with higher pressures and faster rates of change. Each system is activated with posture changes and resets in 1 to 2 days to whatever pressure the body is at, so it is not for long-term control like the renal fluid system.

F. **Chemoreceptors**—detect a decease in O_2 and in increase in CO_2 and H^+. They are several small organs 1 to 2 mm in size, and there are two **carotid bodies** at the bifurcations and several **aortic bodies**. Afferent input from the carotid bodies is to **Hering's nerve** (CN IX) and from the aortic bodies is to the vagus nerve.

G. CNS ischemic response—elicited by an increase in $paCO_2$ detected in the vasomotor center. It is a very powerful sympathetic response and only reacts if the mean arterial pressure is < 60 mm Hg and mainly at 20 mm Hg for emergencies only.

H. Body water—controlled by (1) the anterior hypothalamus with the supraoptic nucleus that secretes ADH to decrease renal H_2O excretion; (2) the lateral hypothalamus that increases H_2O intake by thirst; and (3) the AV-3V region that detects serum osmolarity.

I. Osmolarity receptors—detect an increase in the serum osmolarity and in the serum Na^+ concentration. This causes an increase in ADH secretion that stimulates the loss of Na^+ and other osmolar substrates in the urine and conserves H_2O by decreasing its secretion in the distal tubules. ADH is $\frac{5}{6}$ from the supraoptic nuclei and $\frac{1}{6}$ from the paraventricular nuclei.

J. Serum osmolarity—also controlled by the AV-3V region in the anteroventral third ventricle. The superior part is the **subforniceal organ**, and the inferior part is the **organ vasculosum of the lamina terminalis**. Between these two is the median preoptic nucleus with connections to both the supraoptic nucleus and the BP control centers. There is no BBB here, and the cells act as receptors and shrink if there is an increase in serum Na^+ or a decrease in K^+. They respond by increasing thirst and ADH secretion.

K. Thirst—inhibited by drinking and stomach distention. If there is no change in the serum Na^+, thirst returns in 15 to 30 minutes. It takes 1 hour to absorb the fluid and equalize the osmolarity. If thirst is not stopped before equalization, there may be an overshoot with hyponatremia. The threshold for drinking is reached when the Na^+ rises at least 2 mEq/L above normal or the osmolarity rises 4 mEq/L above normal. The arterial baroreceptors and the atrial volume receptors also increase thirst and ADH secretion.

XXVIII. RESPIRATION

A. The respiratory center—a bilateral center in the medulla and pons.

B. **Dorsal respiratory group**—in the **dorsal medulla** and controls inspiration. It is the **main respiratory center**. Input is from neurons in the nucleus of the solitary tract and also from the chemoreceptors and baroreceptors. There are repetitive inspiratory APs in which one set of neurons fires and inhibits the next. There is a "ramp" signal to the inspiratory muscles with a gradual increase in force followed by complete cessation for 3 seconds and then another cycle. This allows a steady inhalation without gasps.

C. **Ventral respiratory group**—in the **ventrolateral medulla** in the **nucleus ambiguous and retroambiguous**. It controls both **inspiration and expiration**. It is not active in normal breathing when the dorsal nuclear group stimulates inspiration from the diaphragm and the exhalation is by the recoil of the lung and chest. It contributes with the large respiratory efforts from abdominal muscle exhalation and strong inhalation.

D. **Pneumotaxic center**—in the **dorsal superior pons** in the **nucleus parabrachialis** and controls the **rate and pattern of breathing**. It supplies continuous impulses to the inspiratory area to switch it off to shorten a breath and start expiration. Increased input causes rapid breathing and decreased input causes long slow breathing.

E. **Hering-Breuer inflation reflex**—stimulated by stretch receptors in the bronchi and bronchioles. The afferent fibers travel in the vagus nerve to inhibit the dorsal respiratory nucleus to stop respiratory inspiration if the lungs are overly distended. It does not fire until the tidal volume is > 1.5 L (protective function).

F. Chemical control of respiration—used to correct O_2, CO_2, and H^+.

G. Direct control—mediated by CO_2 and H^+. The chemosensitive area of the **ventral medulla** is just below the surface. It excites the respiratory center if there is an **increase in H^+** and less so with an increase in CO_2. The pH has less effect on respiration because H^+ has more affinity for the receptor but does not cross the BBB. CO_2 is a weaker stimulant but crosses the BBB and with H_2O forms HCO_3^- and H^+. The CSF pCO_2 is important because there is little CSF buffering. Changes in $PaCO_2$ are therefore associated with rapid changes in CSF H^+. The response to changes in CO_2 decreases over a few hours to 2 days to $\frac{1}{5}$ of its initial effect, partly by renal clearance of H^+ by increasing the HCO_3^- to bind H^+ in the CSF. PCO_2 causes potent acute respiratory changes but not chronic ones.

H. Indirect control of respiration—by O_2, which does not directly stimulate the respiratory center. The peripheral chemoreceptor system detects O_2, CO_2, and H^+. There are multiple receptors: the carotid bodies travel through Hering's nerve (CN IX) and the aortic bodies travel through CN X, both to the dorsal respiratory area. The carotid and aortic bodies receive special blood flow by means of distinct vessels and because of the large blood flow they always get arterial and not venous blood. It sends increased signals with decreased paO_2 30 to 60 mm Hg as the hemoglobin starts to desaturate. Increased signals are sent with an elevated $paCO_2$ or H^+, but these are seven times weaker than the central receptors, although they are faster. This system probably has little effect on the CO_2 and H^+ control of respiration.

I. During exercise—O_2 use and CO_2 formation increase 20 times. Ventilation increases to keep supply matched to demand. As muscle is stimulated by the brain, collateral fibers go to the respiratory and BP control centers to perform the correct responses (these may be learned). Also joint receptors stimulate respiration. Both chemical and neural factors control respiration, especially with exercise.

XXIX. GASTROINTESTINAL TRACT

A. The GI tract has its own nervous system in the gut wall that extends from the esophagus to the anus and contains 100 million neurons, the same number as the spinal cord. It controls the GI tract movements and secretions.

B. **Auerbach's myenteric plexus**—between the longitudinal and circular layers of muscle and controls GI movements.

C. **Meissner's submucosal plexus**—in the submucosa and controls secretions and blood flow.

D. The sensory nerve endings from the epithelium go to both plexuses, as well as to the sympathetic ganglia, spinal cord, and the parasympathetic fibers in the spinal cord and the brain stem.

E. Parasympathetic system—controls the esophagus to the first half of the colon by means of the vagus nerve. It innervates the sigmoid colon to the anus by way of S2-4. Postganglionic neurons are in the myenteric and submucosal plexuses.

F. Sympathetic system for the GI tract—from T5-L2 and goes to the celiac and mesenteric ganglia to the postganglionic fibers that travel as separate nerves to the intestine's enteric plexus. It acts to decrease movement and smooth muscle contraction (except the muscular mucosa layer).

G. Reflexes—may be (1) entirely enteric; (2) from the intestine to the autonomic system back to the intestine (i.e., the gastrocolic defecation reflex, the enterogastric and colonoileal reflexes to slow transit); and (3) from the intestine to the spinal cord or brain back to the intestine for pain or defecation.

H. Two types of movement in the GI tract:

    1. Propulsive movement—peristalsis. The contractile ring moves forward as a result of stimulation by local reflexcs of distention and irritation and by parasympathetic input. It requires the myenteric plexus to function and moves forward because the plexus is polarized.

    2. Mixing—occurs in the mouth with chewing and in the stomach and intestine as well.

I. Intake—stimulated by hunger. One craves food when the stomach contracts. There may be an appetite for a specific food. The lateral hypothalamus causes the stimulus to eat and increases the emotional drive for food. The ventromedial hypothalamus causes satiety and inhibits the feeding center. There is also control from the amygdala with olfactory input (±) and the prefrontal cortex. The mechanism for intake is in the brain stem and amount of intake is regulated by the hypothalamus. It is stimulated by glucose, amino acid, and lipid levels so nutrient stores can dictate the appetite to achieve long-term control. Appetite decreases with GI distention, CCK (stimulated by the fat in food), glucagon, insulin, and the oral meter of intake with chewing and salivation for short-term control.

J. Obesity—when the nutrient stores do not shut off the hunger center. It may be psychogenic, hypothalamic (different set point of nutrient stores), or genetic.

K. Salivation—controlled by the salivatory nuclei at the medulla/pons junction. The superior nucleus goes to the facial nerve to the submandibular ganglion to the submandibular and sublingual glands. The inferior nucleus goes to CN IX to the otic ganglion to the parotid gland. It is increased by certain tastes (especially sour) and tactile stimulation (increased with smooth and decreased with rough textures). Salivation is controlled by higher areas (increased with disliked food) and gastric stimulation (increased with irritation).

L. Chewing—stimulated by the reticular formation, hypothalamus, amygdala, and cortex with final input into the trigeminal motor nucleus. There is a reflex initiated by a bolus of food that causes the jaw to stretch, and this stimulates the muscles of mastication to contract.

M. Swallowing (deglutition)—voluntary stage with the tongue and involuntary stage from the pharynx through the esophagus. The soft palate pulls up to block the nasal passage, the trachea closes, the esophagus opens, and a fast wave moves the food to the esophagus. The tonsillar pillars have afferent fibers from CN V and IX that go to the solitary tract to the reticular formation swallowing center to CN V, IX, X, XII, and the cervical roots. The esophageal stage has both afferent and efferent fibers from CN X.

N. Gastric secretions—increased with ACh (this increases all secretions: Gastrin, pepsinogen, mucus, HCl), gastrin, and histamine (mainly acid). Acid secretion is by local reflexes (50%) and by the dorsal CN X nucleus to CN X to the enteric system to the gastric glands (50%). The main neurotransmitter is ACh except for gastrin-releasing peptides. Input is from the limbic system and the stomach. It is stimulated by distention of the stomach, tactile sensation in the stomach, and various chemicals (amino acids, peptides, and acids). Increased gastrin secretion is stimulated by the vagus nerve to the parietal cells that produce HCl. Also, gastrin secretion is increased by histamine from the gastric mucosa.

O. Gastric secretions—(1) cephalic phase from the cortex or appetite center in the amygdala or hypothalamus to the dorsal motor nucleus of CN X; (2) gastric phase from vagovagal input, local reflexes, and gastrin release; and (3) intestinal phase mediated by gastrin.

P. Intestinal secretions—mainly controlled by local reflexes. They include mucus to slide feces and electrolyte solutions for absorption and transport.

Q. Defecation—initiated by a stimulus in the rectum. It is controlled by the internal anal sphincter (involuntary smooth muscle) and the external anal sphincter (voluntary striated muscle innervated by the pudendal nerve). The reflex goes to the myenteric plexus to increase peristalsis and relax the sphincters. The urge is increased by the parasympathetic defecation reflex from the pelvic nerves. If one voluntarily counteracts the reflex, it will not occur again until more stool accumulates in the rectum. Sensory fibers can distinguish between gas, liquid, and solid.

XXX. GENITOURINARY TRACT

A. Micturition—involves the bladder's smooth muscle (**detrussor**) and the **internal sphincter**, which are involuntary, and the **external sphincter**, which is voluntary. The parasympathetic system by means of the pelvic nerves from S2 and S3 supply sensation and motor function to the bladder. Stretch is detected by the sensory parasympathetic fibers to the spinal cord to the detrussor for contraction. **The pudendal nerve is for voluntary control to the external sphincter.** There is sympathetic innervation from L2 by way of the hypogastric nerves for pain and blood vessel control but little input for contraction of the bladder and relaxation of the internal sphincter.

B. Micturation reflex—self-regenerating. The initial contraction causes increased sensory input from stretch fibers that causes increased urge and tonic contraction that subsides but increases in frequency until the bladder empties. The reflex is in the spinal cord, but there is upper control by the pons and cortex (both ±) with tonic inhibition and tonic increased tone in the external sphincter. The reflex is initiated by Valsalva's maneuver to increase the stretch reflex. The residual should be less than 10 mL.

C. **Atonic bladder**—caused by decreased sensory input to the spinal cord, so there is overflow incontinence. This is seen with syphilis or LMN injuries.

D. **Spastic bladder**—when there is **no input above the sacrum**. After spinal cord injury, patients have spinal shock without reflexes, so be sure to keep the Foley catheter in or intermittently straight catheterize. When the reflex returns, it may be normal or hyperactive. It may need skin stimulation or suprapubic pressure (Credé's maneuver) for initiation.

XXXI. TEMPERATURE

A. Temperature—autoregulated in dry air 60 to 130°F to keep the body at 97 to 100°F by a hypothalamic-neural mechanism.

B. Detection—by (1) the anterior hypothalamus and preoptic area increases firing mostly with heat, but also with cold, and causes sweating and vasodilation; and (2) the skin and deep tissues have cold (more numerous) and warm receptors. The cold stimulation causes increased shivering to generate heat and decreased sweating and vasoconstriction to conserve heat.

C. Both the anterior hypothalamus and the skin receptors send signals to the posterior hypothalamus to increase heat.

D. Lowering of body temperature—by vasodilation by decreasing sympathetic tone, sweating, and decreasing heat production (decreased shivering and chemical thermogenesis).

E. Raising body temperature—by vasoconstriction, piloerection to increase insulation (sympathetic), increased heat production by shivering, thyroxine to increase the BMR, and increased sympathetic tone. The primary motor center for shivering is in the DM posterior hypothalamus, which is under tonic inhibition by the heat center in the anterior hypothalamus. Stimulation by cold signals from the periphery causes increased body tone and increased heat production five times. Sympathetic input increases cell metabolism for chemical thermogenesis to uncouple oxidative phosphorylation. Body temperature is increased with brown fat that has special mitochondria for heat production (only found in animals and neonates). Body temperature increases with acclimation to cold. Thyroxine causes a delayed increase in cell metabolism, and there are increased levels in chronically cold animals (goiters are more common in a colder climate).

F. Set-point—37°C. Fever results when there is a change in the set-point by proteins, chemicals, or toxins called pyrogens. Gram-negative bacterial endotoxin is taken up by WBCs; this causes increased **IL-1**, which causes increased prostaglandins, which cause fever from the hypothalamus in 8 hours. Treat by blocking the prostaglandin formation with aspirin. Fevers may also be caused by tumors or surgery near the hypothalamus.

XXXII. ENDOCRINE

A. Pituitary gland—secretes eight hormones, six from the anterior pituitary and two from the posterior pituitary gland.

B. Hypothalamus—gathers information (pain, smells, electrolytes, etc.) and relays it to the pituitary gland.

C. The primary capillary plexus of the median eminence of the hypothalamus and the tuber cinereum drain to the hypothalamic-hypophyseal portal system with sinuses to the anterior pituitary gland.

D. The hypothalamic cell bodies are diffusely spread out, but the axons go to the median eminence. The hypothalamus secretes releasing and inhibiting hormones: TRH, CRH, GHRH, and GHIH (somatostatin), GnRH, and PIF (DA). Somatostatin inhibits GHRH and TRH.

E. All anterior pituitary hormones except GH work on target organs.

F.

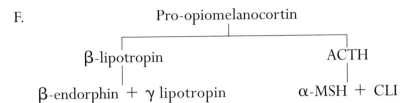

Pro-opiomelanocortin

β-lipotropin   ACTH

β-endorphin + γ lipotropin   α-MSH + CLI

G. Growth hormone (GH)—promotes infant-to-child and child-to-adult growth by increasing bone and tissue growth. Bones stop growing when the cells in the epiphysis are used up. It also has metabolic functions, such as increasing protein formation and fat use and decreasing carbohydrate use. Somatomedin C is synthesized in the liver in response to GH, acts on the end organs, and helps provide feedback by increasing the level of somatostatin and decreasing GH. A deficiency early in life causes dwarfism. An excess early in life causes giantism and later in life causes acromegaly.

H. Thyroid-stimulating hormone (TSH)—increases the rate of body metabolism and heat production. Hypothyroidism early in life causes cretinism.

I. Andrenocorticotropin hormone (ACTH)—stimulates the production of cortisol to react to stress. It also stimulates aldosterone, which is more controlled by K^+, Na^+, and angiotensin. It decreases protein formation and increases metabolism (using amino acids elsewhere to repair damage or as energy to make carbohydrates). It increases fat and glucose use.

J. Prolactin (PR)—increases with pregnancy and causes an increase in fetal protein growth, increase in breast size, and increase in milk secretions after pregnancy (inhibited by estrogen and progesterone before birth). It is stimulated by sucking through a spinal cord reflex. It is tonically inhibited by PIF (DA). Stress may decrease the secretion of PR and cause a mother to stop secreting milk.

K. Leutinizing hormone (LH) increases Leydig's cell's testosterone production and hyperplasia.

L. Follicular stimulating hormone (FSH) and LH—increased by warm weather and more light in the day. This correlates with the time of the year when mating often is productive and offspring have the best chance of survival. There is also psychic input so that stress can decrease fertility. Testosterone inhibits the hypothalamic GnRH so it decreases LH secretion. Spermatogenesis by the testes causes Sertoli's cells to secrete inhibin to decrease FSH by the anterior pituitary to inhibit the Sertoli's cells to prevent overproduction. Sertoli's cells provide nutrition to the developing sperm. Puberty occurs around age 13. GnRH is not secreted in childhood, before puberty. This may be by amygdala input to the hypothalamus.

M. Female sexual response—GnRH is secreted mainly by the arcuate nucleus in the medial basal hypothalamus with input from the limbic system (psychogenic). Low estrogen levels and high progesterone levels decrease the FSH/LH secretion mainly at the anterior pituitary gland but also at the hypothalamus. Inhibin secreted by the corpus luteum (CL) decreases FSH and some LH secretion (may end cycle). There are increased LH levels 48 hours before ovulation (also a slight increase in FSH).

1. In the first half of the cycle, estrogen will actually have a positive feedback and increase the FSH/LH. Also progesterone by the CL may increase the LH surge for ovulation.

2. After ovulation, the CL increases the level of progesterone, estrogen, and inhibin to decrease FSH/LH. Three days before menstruation, the CL involutes and decreases the estrogen and progesterone secretion to cause an increase in FSH/LH and menstruation.

3. The peak estrogen level is at 13 days after the start of menstruation. Twelve days after the onset of menstruation, the FSH and LH that were slowly decreased by estrogen's negative feedback increase significantly by positive feedback to increase the LH and the FSH surge for ovulation and CL formation.

4. Menarche—occurs at 13 years. Menopause occurs at 40 to 50 years. There is decreased estrogen production by ovarian burnout, so there is no inhibition or surge of FSH and LH.

5. The female sexual response requires psychic and local stimulation. There is increased desire at ovulation with the peak level of estrogen.

   (a) Input—from the pudendal nerve to the spinal cord and brain.

   (b) Output—by means of the sacral plexus to the nervi erigentes of the parasympathetic system to the erectile tissue of the clitoris. It also tightens the vagina around the penis to increase pleasure for both.

   (c) There is increased Bartholin's gland secretion of mucus under the labia minora. Fluid is also secreted by the vaginal wall and by the male.

   (d) The sympathetic system is involved in the orgasm, which helps promote fertilization by increasing the uterus and fallopian tube motility and increasing cervical dilation. It also causes perineal contraction and an increased oxytocin production to increase the uterine contraction. This way it facilitates sperm transport to the uterus.

N. Male sexual response—involves afferent fibers from the pudendal nerves to the sacral plexus to the spinal cord to the brain. Irritation or full sensation of the sexual organs causes increased sexual desire (aphrodisiac).

   1. The sexual act is completely coded in spinal reflexes (input above the lumbar level is not needed), although psychic factors can influence it.

   2. Parasympathetic input—causes an erection (remember the "p" in point) because the spinal cord by way of the nervi erigentes supplies the penis to cause an increase in blood flow.

   3. There is increased mucus secreted by the urethra and bulbourethral glands for some lubrication.

   4. Sympathetic input—causes ejaculation (remember the "s" in shoot) from the L1 and 2 levels to the hypogastric and pelvic plexi. Emission is from the vas deferens and ampulla contracting to push the sperm out to the urethra. The prostate with muscle contraction and the seminal vesicle provide the fluid to form sperm and mixes with the urethral mucus.

5. Ejaculation—when there is fullness sensed by the pudendal nerves that go to the spinal cord that causes contraction of all genital organs and the ischiocavernosus and bulbocavernosus rhythmically. It also stimulates pelvic thrusts.

O. Posterior pituitary gland—secretes oxytocin and ADH, which are synthesized in the cell bodies of the supraoptic and paraventricular nuclei of the hypothalamus, coupled to neurophysins (carrier proteins), placed in vesicles, and transported along the axons to the posterior pituitary gland, where they can be identified as Herring bodies.

P. ADH—secreted when an increase in the osmolarity or Na^+ is detected by the receptors in the supraoptic nucleus. It causes increased **distal tubule** H_2O resorption and NaCl loss. Most $\left(\frac{5}{6}\right)$ is secreted from the supraoptic nucleus and the rest by the paraventricular nucleus. Its release is stimulated by warm skin, vomiting, decreased blood volume, pain, narcotics, and angiotensin 2. Its release is decreased by ETOH and cold. CRH inhibits ADH.

Q. Oxytocin—mostly secreted by the paraventricular nucleus $\left(\frac{5}{6}\right)$. It causes uterine contraction at the end of pregnancy. Secretion is increased with cervical stimulation for positive feedback. Sucking causes oxytocin secretion that causes the myoepithelial cells in the breast glands to contract and excrete milk.

Glossary

A

ACA	anterior cerebral artery
ACh	acetylcholine
ACOM	anterior communicating artery
ACTH	adrenocorticotropic hormone
ADH	antidiuretic hormone
AFP	alpha-fetoprotein
AICA	anterior inferior cerebellar artery
AIDS	acquired immune deficiency syndrome
ALL	anterior longitudinal ligament
AMPA	2-(aminoethyl)phenylacetic acid
AP	anteroposterior; action potential
APUD	amine precursor uptake and decarboxylation
ARAS	ascending reticular activating system
ATIII	antithrombin III
ATPase	adenosine triphosphatase
ATP	adenosine triphosphatase
AV	atrioventricular
AVM	arteriovenous malformation

B

BAER	brain stem auditory evoked response
BBB	blood-brain barrier
BMR	basal metabolic rate
BP	blood pressure
BT	bleeding time
BUN	blood urea nitrogen

C

CAI	complete androgen insensitivity
CAM	cell adhesion molecule
CAMP	cyclic adenosine monophosphate

CBC	complete blood count
CBF	cerebral blood flow
CCA	common carotid artery
CCK	cholecystokinin
CEA	carcinoembryonic antigen
cGMP	cyclic guanosine monophosphate
CHF	congestive heart failure
CK	creatine kinase
CL	centralis lateralis; corpus luteum
CM	centromedial
CMRO$_2$	cerebral metabolic rate of oxygen
CN	cranial nerve
CNS	central nervous system
CO	cardiac output
CoA	coenzyme A
COP	colloid osmotic pressure
CPA	cerebellopontine angle
CPM	central pontine myelinosis
CRH	corticotropin-releasing hormone
CSF	cerebrospinal fluid
CT	computed tomography
CVA	cerebrovascular accident

D

D	diopter
DA	dopamine
DAG	diacylglycerol
DAI	diffuse axonal injury
DDAVP	desmopressin acetate
DDI	dideoxyinosine
DI	diabetes insipidus
DIC	disseminated intravascular coagulation

DLF	dorsal longitudinal fasciculus
DM	dorsomedial
DMSO	dimethyl sulfoxide
DNA	deoxyribonucleic acid
DOPA	dihydroxyphenylalanine (methyldopa)
DPG	2,3-diphosphoglycerate
DRG	dorsal root ganglion
DSC	dorsal spinocerebellar
DTR	deep tendon reflex
DVT	deep venous thrombosis

E

ECA	external carotid artery
EC-IC	external carotid-internal carotid
EDTA	ethylenediaminetetraacetic acid
EEG	electroencephalogram
EHL	extensor hallucis longus
EMG	electromyelogram
EPI	epinephrine
EPSP	excitatory postsynaptic potential
ER	endoplasmic reticulum
ESR	erythrocyte sedimentation rate
ET	endotracheal
ETOH	ethanol

F

FE	fractional excretion
FFH1	Forel's field H1 (thalamic fasciculus)
FFH2	Forel's field H2 (lenticular fasciculus)
FFP	fresh frozen plasma
FSH	follicle-stimulating hormone

G

GABA	gamma-aminobutyric acid
GBM	glioblastoma multiforme
GCS	Glasgow coma scale
GDP	guanosine diphosphate
GFAP	glial fibrillary acidic protein
GH	growth hormone

GHIH	growth hormone-inhibiting hormone
GHRH	growth hormone-releasing hormone
GI	gastrointestinal
GnRH	gonadotropin-releasing hormone
GP	globus pallidus
GPe	globus pallidus externa
GPm	medial globus pallidus
GPi	globus pallidus interna
GSA	general somatic afferent
GSE	general somatic efferent
GTP	guanosine triphosphate
GU	genitourinary
GVA	general visceral afferent
GVE	general visceral efferent

H

Hb	hemoglobin
HCG	human chorionic gonadotropin
HDL	high-density lipoprotein
HGPRT	hypoxanthine-guanine phosphoribosyltransferase
HIV	human immunodeficiency virus
HLA-DR2	human leukocyte antigen-DR2
HMB	homatropine methylbromide
5-HT	5-hydroxytryptamine (serotonin)
HTLV	human T-cell lymphotropic virus

I

IC	internal capsule
ICA	internal carotid artery
ICAM	intercellular adhesion molecule
ICH	intracranial hemorrhage
ICP	intracranial pressure
IFN	interferon
Ig	immunoglobulin
IL	interleukin
IM	intramuscular
INO	internuclear ophthalmoplegia
IP_3	inositol 1,4,5-triphosphate

IPSP	inhibitory postsynaptic potential		MRI	magnetic resonance imaging
IQ	intelligence quotient		MS	multiple sclerosis
ITP	idiopathic thrombocytopenic purpura		MSG	monosodium glutamate
IV	intravenous		MSH	melanocyte-stimulating hormone
IVDA	intravenous drug abuse		MXT	methotrexate

J

JGA — juxtaglomerular apparatus

L

LD — lateral dorsal
LDH — lactate dehydrogenase
LE — lower extremity
LGB — lateral geniculate body
LH — luteinizing hormone
LHRH — luteinizing hormone-releasing hormone
LMN — lower motor neuron
LOAF — lumbricals 1 and 2, opponens pollicis, and abductor and flexor pollicis brevis
LP — lateral posterior; lumbar puncture

M

MAO — monoamine oxidase
MBP — myelin basic protein
MCA — middle cerebral artery
MCP — metacarpophalangeal
MD — mediodorsal; muscular dystrophy
MEPP — miniature end-plate potential
MFB — medial forebrain bundle
MG — myasthenia gravis
MGB — medial geniculate body
MI — myocardial infarction
ML — medial lemniscus
MLF — medial longitudinal fasciculus
MM — multiple myeloma
MOF — multiple organ failure
MPNST — malignant peripheral nerve sheath tumor
MPS — mucopolysaccharides
MRA — magnetic resonance angiography

N

NAC — N-acetylcysteine
NAPA — N-acetylprocainamide
NCV — nerve conduction velocity
NE — norepinephrine
NMDA — N-methyl-D-aspartate
NMJ — neuromuscular junction
NREM — nonrapid eye movement
NS — normal saline
NSAID — nonsteroidal anti-inflammatory drug

O

OCP — oral contraceptive pill
OPLL — ossified posterior longitudinal ligament

P

PAM — L-phenylalanine mustard (melphalan)
PAS — periodic acid–Schiff
PCA — posterior cerebral artery
PCOM — posterior communicating artery
PCR — polymerase chain reaction
PCV — procarbazine, CCNU (lomustine), vincristine
PF — parafasciculus
Pi — protease inhibitor
PICA — posterior inferior cerebellar artery
PIF — prolactin-inhibiting hormone
PKU — phenylketonuria
PLL — posterior longitudinal ligament
PMN — polymorphonuclear neutrophils
PNS — peripheral nervous system
PPRF — paramedian pontine reticular formation
PR — prolactin
PRBCs — packed red blood cells

PT	prothrombin time
PTAH	phosphotungstic acid hematoxylin
PTH	parathyroid hormone
PTT	partial thromboplastin time
PTU	propylthiouracil
PVR	peripheral vascular resistance

R

RA	rheumatoid arthritis
RBC	red blood cell
RBF	renal blood flow
REM	rapid eye movement
REZ	root entry zone
RF	radiofrequency
RiMLF	rostral interstitial nucleus of the MLF
RIND	reversible ischemic neurologic deficit
RMP	resting membrane potential

S

SA	special afferent; sinoatrial
SAH	subarachnoid hemorrhage
SBP	systolic blood pressure
SCA	superior cerebellar artery
SDH	subdural hematoma
SI	substantia innominata; sacroiliac
SIADH	syndrome of inappropriate antidiuretic hormone (secretion)
SL	sublingual
SLE	systemic lupus erythematosus
SMA	spinal muscle atrophy
SN	substantia nigra
SNpc	substantia nigra pars compacta
SNpr	substantia nigra pars reticulata
SQ	subcutaneous
SR	sarcoplasmic reticulum
SSA	special somatic afferent
SSEP	somatosensory evoked potential

SSPE	subacute sclerosing panencephalitis
ST	subthalamus
SVC	superior vena cava
SVE	special visceral efferent
SVR	systemic vascular resistance

T

T_3	triiodothyronine
T_4	thyroxine
TBG	thyroid-binding globulin
TBW	total body water
TCL	transverse carpal ligament
TEA	tetraethylammonium
TENS	transcutaneous electrical nerve stimulation
TIA	transient ischemic attack
TMJ	temporomandibular joint
TNF	tumor necrosis factor
tPA	tissue plasminogen activator
TRH	thyroid-releasing hormone
tRNA	transfer ribonucleic acid
TSH	thyroid-stimulating hormone
TTP	thrombotic thrombocytopenic purpura

U

UE	upper extremity
UMN	upper motor neuron

V

VA	ventroanterior; visceral afferent
VEP	visual evoked potential
VL	ventrolateral
VPI	ventral posterior inferior
VPL	ventroposterolateral
VPM	ventroposteromedial
vWF	von Willebrand's factor

W

WBC	white blood cell

Figure Acknowledgments

ANATOMY

Figure 1 "Copyright, 1997. Icon Learning Systems, LLC, a subsidiary of Havas MediMedia USA Inc. Reprinted with permission from ICON Learning Systems, LLC, illustrated by Frank H. Netter, MD. All rights reserved."

Figure 2 Illustration by Lydia M. Johns.

Figure 3 *Microneurosurgery I*. Yasargil MG. New York, NY: Thieme, 1984. (Figure 123)

Figure 7 (Top) Illustration by Lydia M. Johns.

Figure 7 (Bottom) "Copyright, 1997. Icon Learning Systems, LLC, a subsidiary of Havas MediMedia USA Inc. Reprinted with permission from ICON Learning Systems, LLC, illustrated by Frank H. Netter, MD. All rights reserved."

Figure 8 (Top) Illustration by Lydia M. Johns.

Figure 8 (Bottom) "Copyright, 1997. Icon Learning Systems, LLC, a subsidiary of Havas MediMedia USA Inc. Reprinted with permission from ICON Learning Systems, LLC, illustrated by Frank H. Netter, MD. All rights reserved."

Figure 9 *Microneurosurgery I*. Yasargil MG. New York, NY: Thieme, 1984. (Figure 117)

Figures 10–11 "Copyright, 1997. Icon Learning Systems, LLC, a subsidiary of Havas MediMedia USA Inc. Reprinted with permission from ICON Learning Systems, LLC, illustrated by Frank H. Netter, MD. All rights reserved."

Figure 12 *Neurosurgery Board Review*. Alleyne Jr. CH. New York, NY: Thieme, 1997. (Figure 161)

Figures 13–15 "Copyright, 1997. Icon Learning Systems, LLC, a subsidiary of Havas MediMedia USA Inc. Reprinted with permission from ICON Learning Systems, LLC, illustrated by Frank H. Netter, MD. All rights reserved."

Figure 16 Illustration by Lydia M. Johns.

Figure 18 *Human Anatomy 2*. Frick H, Leonhardt H, Starck D. New York, NY: Thieme, 1991. (Figure 118)

Figure 19 *Human Anatomy 2*. Frick H, Leonhardt H, Starck D. New York, NY: Thieme, 1991. (Figure 119)

Figure 20 *Human Anatomy 2*. Frick H, Leonhardt H, Starck D. New York, NY: Thieme, 1991. (Figure 110)

Figure 21 *Human Anatomy 2*. Frick H, Leonhardt H, Starck D. New York, NY: Thieme, 1991. (Figure 111)

Figure 22 *Human Anatomy 2*. Frick H, Leonhardt H, Starck D. New York, NY: Thieme, 1991. (Figure 139)

Figure 23 Illustration by Lydia M. Johns.

Figure 24 *Human Anatomy 2*. Frick H, Leonhardt H, Starck D. New York, NY: Thieme, 1991. (Figure 142)

Figures 25–28 Illustration by Lydia M. Johns.

Figures 29A-D *Color Atlas / Text of Human Anatomy. Volume 3: Nervous System and Sensory Organs*. Kahle W, Leonhardt H, Platzer W. New York, NY: Thieme, 1993. (Page 217)

Figures 29 E-G *Color Atlas / Text of Human Anatomy. Volume 3: Nervous System and Sensory Organs*. Kahle W, Leonhardt H, Platzer W. New York, NY: Thieme, 1993. (Page 219)

Figure 31 Illustration by Lydia M. Johns.

Figure 32 *Human Anatomy 2*. Frick H, Leonhardt H, Starck D. New York, NY: Thieme, 1991. (Figure 98)

Figure 33 *Human Anatomy 2*. Frick H, Leonhardt H, Starck D. New York, NY: Thieme, 1991. (Figure 105)

Figures 34–40 Illustration by Lydia M. Johns.

Figure 41 *Human Anatomy 2*. Frick H, Leonhardt H, Starck D. New York, NY: Thieme, 1991. (Figure 95)

Figure 42 *Human Anatomy 2*. Frick H, Leonhardt H, Starck D. New York, NY: Thieme, 1991. (Figure 96)

Figure 43 *Human Anatomy 2*. Frick H, Leonhardt H, Starck D. New York, NY: Thieme, 1991. (Figure 133)

Figures 44–52 "Copyright, 1997. Icon Learning Systems, LLC, a subsidiary of Havas MediMedia USA Inc. Reprinted with permission from ICON Learning Systems, LLC, illustrated by Frank H. Netter, MD. All rights reserved."

Figures 53–54 Illustration by Lydia M. Johns.

Figures 55–56 "Copyright, 1997. Icon Learning Systems, LLC, a subsidiary of Havas MediMedia USA Inc. Reprinted with permission from ICON Learning Systems, LLC, illustrated by Frank H. Netter, MD. All rights reserved."

Figures 58–62 Illustration by Lydia M. Johns.

Figure 62 *Human Anatomy 2*. Frick H, Leonhardt H, Starck D. New York, NY: Thieme, 1991. (Figure 179)

PHYSIOLOGY

Figure 1 *Human Anatomy 2*. Frick H, Leonhardt H, Starck D. New York, NY: Thieme, 1991. (Figure 159)

Figures 2A,B *Human Anatomy 2*. Frick H, Leonhardt H, Starck D. New York, NY: Thieme, 1991. (Figures 167 and 168)

Figure 3 *Human Anatomy 2*. Frick H, Leonhardt H, Starck D. New York, NY: Thieme, 1991. (Figure 165)

Figures 5–8 Illustration by Lydia M. Johns.

Index